Surgical Sutures

A Practical Guide of Surgical Knots and Suturing Techniques Used in Emergency Rooms, Surgery, and General Medicine

Nathan Orwell

Copyright © 2021 _ Nathan Orwell

Disclaimer

All the information in this book is to be used for informational and educational purposes only. The author will not, in any way, account for any results that stem from the use of the contents herein. While conscious and creative attempts have been made to ensure that all information provided herein is as accurate and useful as possible, the author is not legally bound to be responsible for any damage caused by the accuracy as well as the use/misuse of this information.

Table of Contents

INTRODUCTION

Many students are bothered with understanding this phase of their training and having to cope with the practice afterward. No qualms. You can easily understand the subject of "suture" by simply going through this material carefully.

The word "suture" is a medical terminology often used to describe a stitch or stitches done to secure apposition or fit together wound areas in any part of the body. The wounds could be traumatic or surgical; induced by the use of specialized medical instruments. So, what is used to ensure this is called "suture materials." These are artificial fibers that ensure the coupling of the wounded regions or cut areas.

Historical View

History has it that suturing has existed for a long time, and different artificial fibers or threads have been developed. It is being used by the likes of surgeons, psychiatrists, and nurses for the same course. It is important to take note of the practice of suturing, which is dated as far back as 3000 BC amongst the ancient Egyptians. Let's introduce you to some historical facts about the practice of suturing and its materials. It is evidenced that "eyed needles" made of bones were used for the same process at the onset. Some other materials used then were hair, grass, reeds, pig bristles, cotton, needles built with different materials such as copper, silver, and bone, amongst many.

Today, with the advent of technology, many modernized and sophisticated instruments ensure a proper suturing process. Different sutures repair different wounds; hence, the surgeon or medical professional must understand what necessitates the use of different types of sutures. Having known that there are different types of sutures, under normal circumstances, the practice should be tolerable to some changes in the wound, such as swelling. Also, to minimize inflammation and be inexpensive. However, not all of these qualities are found in a particular type of suture, which means that one has to understand the peculiarities in order to be confident of what type of suture to be administered when the surgeon is faced with different types of wounds.

That is a very important practice that must be learned by every medical student, most especially those that are specialized in surgery. It requires some specified techniques to be carried out under an aseptic or sterile condition and sophisticated equipment.

Contrary to the general opinion of beginners in medicine, where it is believed that suturing is only for holding open tissues together, it is in the best interest of every medical student to know that beyond this common opinion, it has in its pocket other purposes. While the focus of suturing is to foster healing, it is important to see this healing process as both primary and secondary. Further to the importance of suturing is that it assists in the process of hemostasis by covering a bleeding region of the wounded part of the body. It likewise ensures anastomosis by redirecting blood to another part asides from that injured region. It also ensures low dehiscence rates and stronger tensile strength. In addition, it makes access to tissues visible and convenient and ensures the repair of tendons and nerves at the wounded or injured area of the body.

Like in every practice, as there is a simple phase, there is also the complicated or more advanced side. Such is what you should expect in the practice of suturing as a medical professional. With this in mind, every medical professional, most especially surgeons, must be circumspect with how they suture as it's very critical in surgery. If not properly done, it would lead to postoperative complications. Some of these complications are infection, wound deterioration, presence of scars. Therefore, beyond doubt, it is expected of every student to pursue the thorough practice of suturing and become skillful in conducting it.

Having been introduced to the subject of "suture" and its importance, you should be aware of what this book will avail you, which are: History of wound care and sutures, aseptic techniques in suturing, armamentarium, surgical needles, and hand instrument, blades and its types, surgical knots comprising properties of an ideal knot, the principles of tying knots, and different types of knots, not forgetting process of wound and bone healing as it is important for a surgeon to detect early the indications of an infected or not so good wound. Also, you would get to learn the different types of sutures, various techniques of suturing, how sloppy hands can be managed, which comes with quick exercises.

It is certain that as soon as you're done with this book, you'll be excited to share it with the next available medical student or professional you know.

History of Wound Care

While the term wound has been common among people since the olden days, in the sense that you will be hearing, "I'm wounded, or I'm injured," still many people are yet to grab the origin and how the word wound came into place. The term wound was initially called *"wund,"* meaning hurt, injury, or ulcer; an injury to living tissue. It's fantastic to know that some of the principles of wound care have been known since 2000BC. When wound care history is mentioned, this is entirely the history of human beings because, without humans, there won't be any wounds; talk less of how to take care of them. So, a wound is as old as time humans. Among the oldest manuscripts of medicine known to humans is the clay tablet that has been in use since 2200BC. The tablet features a description of the three healing gestures known as; washing the wounds, making the plasters, and bandaging the wounds. Even in the olden days' medicine, they have many fantastic healing techniques that will always keep one wondering. It will also amaze you to know that the olden days' plasters are still what medical personnel use in the present days for wound dressing. The plasters consist of many important things, including mud, clay, plants, and herbs. These plasters aim to provide coverage and protection to the wounds and absorb exudate from the wounds. During those days, an important and common ingredient used in plasters was oil. Surely, a wound can get some protection from oil because bacteria hardly grow in the oil. Another important benefit of the oil is that it prevents the bandage from sticking to the wound, serving as a non-adherent dressing.

Another amazing wound care ingredient or item in the olden days was beer, which is known among the Sumerians. These people can brew a minimum of 19 different types of beer. Also, there was this amazing wound healing prescription known in Mesopotamian culture which states, "Pound together, fur-turpentine, pine-turpentine, tamarisk, daisy, and flour of inninnu strain, all mixed in milk and beer in a small copper pan, then spread on the skin; bind on hom and he shall recover." The Egyptians were the first to use honey for healing. The Egyptians commonly use honey, grease, and lint to make their plasters. While honey may be seen as an antibacterial agent, it has some wound care properties, which are still used in present-day medicine. Long before the time of Christ, the Indian people had been using honey as a wound care agent. The Egyptians regard the color green as an indication of life, so they always paint their wound green, and it's well known that green contains copper. While most people think of the pyramids and mummies when Ancient Egypt is mentioned, their art of wrapping the bodies of the dead always influenced the art of bandaging the wound, which doubles its importance by providing protection against the spread of infection.

Coming back to the Greeks, they always stress the importance and benefits of cleanliness in the sense that they always recommend boiling clean water with vinegar and wine and washing a wound with it. Another amazing thing known with the Greeks is they can differentiate between a fresh, concealing, and a chronic wound. Back to the Hippocratic collection on wound healing, an expert stated, "for an obstinate ulcer, using sweet wine and a lot of patients should be enough for healing." The Romans regard four cardinal signs of inflammation as an important art of medicine; redness, swelling, heat, and pain.

Back to the topic in hand, in the 18th century, surgery was regarded as an important and respected branch of medicine, moving to the 19th century when antiseptic techniques got great recognition and breakthrough which provided great advancement in the field of medicine, especially with the introduction of antibiotics which provide a great benefit in controlling infection and decreasing mortality.

The modern aspect of healing came into place in the 20th century. With technological advancement, more than thousands of healing products globally contain highly absorbent materials such as alginates, foams, and carboxymethylcellulose. Everything changed in the aspect of medicine, such as the invention of occlusive dressing and semi-occlusive dressing, growth factors, advanced honey-based dressing, and a lot of methods to treat acute or chronic wounds.

And still, there was the invention of sutures in the aspect of healing, also called stitches. Sutures have also been known for thousands of years. Since this book focuses on sutures, below is an explicit discussion on the history of sutures, how they came into existence, the dates, and who first performed suturing.

History of Sutures

When explaining everything in the life of humans, history has to come into play, especially in the aspect of medicine and surgery.

History has it that suturing has existed for a long time, and different artificial fibers or threads have been developed. It is being used by the likes of surgeons, psychiatrists, and nurses for the same course. It is important to understand that the practice of suturing is dated as far back as 3000 BC amongst the ancient Egyptians. Let's introduce you to some historical facts about the practice of suturing and its materials. It is evidenced that "eyed needles" made of bones were used for the same process at the onset. Some other materials used then were hair, grass, reeds, pig bristles, cotton, needles built with different materials such as copper, silver, and bone, amongst many.

It is known that surgeons held suturing tools, knives, and cautery in their possession for many years. The greatness of sutures didn't stop there; basic and complex surgeries became easier with sutures. Even though only a few surgeons understand that behind the familiar foil packaging, a great and awesome history exists. While it's impossible to describe all the important papers associated with the history of sutures, knowing some important and excellent descriptions by surgeons and scientists will greatly benefit you. We'll be getting to that shortly.

The important tools and equipment used for today's sutures were results of great practice and experience from many centuries back. Some materials mentioned above, like the hair, tendon, wool, and threads found in mummified remains, were used by Egyptians for sutures. Edwith Smith (1822-1906), a great surgeon, discovered a papyrus of medical knowledge certified in 1600 BCE. The papyrus bearing the name Smith is a roll of more than 15ft long containing more than 500 lines of text, coupled with over 40 illustrations concerning medical treatments and trauma. This piece became an important piece in the history of medicine and civilization. Being the oldest known surgical text, it is currently on a long-term loan from the New York Academy of medicine to the New York Metropolis Museum of Art. In the papyrus, the suture was mentioned and described in detail. An example of a detailed treatment of laceration is written in the papyrus, "If thou findest that wound open and its stitching loosed, thou shouldn't draw together for him the gash with two strips of linen." The Egyptian embalmers use this method to stitch up a corpse after removing an organ.

Indian surgeon Susruta wrote the first document talking about the suturing technique known as *Samhita* in 500 BCE. Susruta described many beneficial healing procedures, including the use of large black ants in the margins of wounds, writing that the insect jaws will effectively staple the incision shut.

Susruta also detailed the use of bowstring made from sheep upper small intestine as a suturing technique for rhinoplasty, tonsillectomy, amputation, and repair of anal fistula. Back then, catgut was available from musicians who used material for stringed instruments.

After 200 years, Hippocrates and his disciples revived the logic of medical thinking and teaching in ancient Greece. These ancient people contributed greatly to the surgical and medical aspects.

Aurelius Cornelius Celsus, a Roman medical journalist and teacher, wrote the 8th volume of the *De Re Medicina,* which describes the use of braided sutures and is currently in use, especially in ligature for hemostasis. Celsus wrote about controlling hemostasis by "making ligature in many places." Twisting around the vessels. He also describes some signs and symptoms of infection as calor, tumor, rubor, and dolor, which are also currently in use in many medical schools.

Galen Pergamon (131-211) was also the first person to describe the use of gut string as a suture material to stitch severed tendons in gladiators. Like the former scientists, Galen also recommended some procedures for the closure of wounds by using sutures; copious irrigation of wounds with diluted wine. He also recommended using silk sutures. Galen's teaching remains of great benefit and centuries after his death.

Cautery became the standard for wound hemostasis during the 8th century. Heated oils were also used for bleeding wounds and vessels, but this also can cause severe damage to the tissues around the wounded area.

Many other surgeons made a great contribution in the aspect of medicine within this time, including Rhazes (850-923) from Baghdad, a surgeon who continued to use the cat guy lute string for the repair of the abdominal wall.

After the death of Rhazes, it came to Ali Ibn Sinna ([980-1037], popularly known as Avicenna), notice that the sutures were rapidly dissolved due to infection of an anal fistula. While searching for more pronounced suturing materials, Avicenna discovered a natural monofilament structure, pig's bristles in the *Canon of Medicine.* He also demonstrates the use of a loop of sutures for abdominal closure, avoiding the weakest part of a suture which is the knot.

At the same time, Abulcasis (936 CE) also describes a detailed explanation of cautery. Working together with Avicenna, at that time, Abulcasis was working on cautery subjugated suture technique.

The preceding knowledge was kept by monasteries while monks translated and copied the text.

Around the 5th-15th centuries, there was a small medical innovation. There was also a little change during the 16th-18th century made by a Frenchman surgeon called Ambroise Paré, who avoided cauterizing the opening of wounds with boiling oil and reintroduced Galen, Celsus, and Avicenna methods to be used after limb amputation. Paré also warned about leaving dead space shallow when closing a wound. He also used fine linen strips and silk for vascular ligatures. Peré has a popular motor, "Je le pansy,

Dieu le guarit," meaning "I tended his wound; God cured him."

Philip Syng Physick (1768-1837), an American physician, brought about detailed knowledge on the absorption properties of suture materials. He was a lecturer in Philadelphia Medical Schools. He was also the first professor at the University of Pennsylvania who discovered that the fluid that escaped from wounds dissolved leather. He also found that ligatures that dissolved the wound would be helpful. Although his published books were minimal, they play an important role in today's medicine. Physick used chronic sutures and also made them popular.

James Marion Sims (1813-1884) also popularized the use of silver wire for vesicovaginal fistulas. Sims discovered that inflammation causes usage of chronic and silk to repair fistula to fail. He described the use of silver wire in 1853, during *Anniversary Discourse* to the New York Academy of Medicine. Sims developed many things that provided great advances in medicine, including the successful treatment of vesicovaginal fistula after many failed attempts from some surgeons.

He used needle drivers to pass sutures through tissue retractors to place his sutures for vesicovaginal fistula repair.

Nowadays, many suturing materials are used, and some of the olden days' materials are modernized.

The use of sutures became globally known around the 19th century, but a problem arose due to the discovery of infection in sutured wounds or infection. As a result, many surgeons of that era preferred to cauterize wounds than risk their patients' lives due to infection.

Lord Joseph Lister's (1867) discovery made a great contribution to the advancement of suture techniques. In his publication titled "*The Antiseptic System*," he observed the suppuration condition and made some connections between germs' presence and infection. Before his discovery, sutures were left due to infection. He described that if the suturing instruments can be kept clean by eliminating the bacteria, with the end cut short, the materials can be left *in situ*. During his first human experiment, he observed that healing could take place without any suppuration and with the absence of swelling or tenderness. He used some materials, including carbolic acid, to clean all his suturing materials. Advancement in sutured sterilization continued to be achieved with time.

To date, the majority of the discoveries of all the physicians are modernized and put to use.

Aseptic Techniques in Suturing Procedure

Surgeons and overall medical professionals use aseptic techniques method to protect their patients from infection.

The word aseptic or asepsis refers to the absence of germs that can cause disease or infection.

It is generally known that the skin is the first line of defense against surrounding infection in a situation where there is a break in the skin either because of injury caused by accident or surgical infection. Aseptic techniques help in preventing the body from healthcare-associated infections (HCAIs). These healthcare-associated infections are infections that patients develop as a result of treatments from medical professionals.

Common healthcare-associated infections include:

- **Catheter-associated urinary tract infections:** This occurs when a catheter is inserted into a patient. It is characterized by the transfer of germs along the catheter, which can cause infection in the bladder or kidney.

- **Central line-associated bloodstream infection:** This type of infection occurs when germs like bacteria or viruses enter the bloodstream through the central.

- **Clostridium difficile infection:** This is an infection caused by the bacteria clostridium difficile that occurs in the colon.

- **Surgical site infection:** This is an unwanted infection that occurs in the incision, which is created by an invasive surgical procedure that causes hospital mobility, doubles mortality, and increases the length of stay in the hospital.

- **Ventilator-associated pneumonia:** This is characterized by the development of pneumonia two or more days after mechanical ventilation administered by using an endotracheal tube or tracheotomy. The infection occurs due to the inversion of microorganisms in the lower respiratory tract and parenchyma.

Infections like the ones mentioned above are an important concern in the healthcare community. These infections can lead to severe complications for the affected individual and cause disciplinary consequences for the medical facilities.

Aseptic techniques are classified into many categories, including simple practices like using alcohol, full surgical asepsis like using sterile gowns, gloves, and masks.

Nowadays, many healthcare facilities use aseptic techniques in their practice, especially in places like surgery rooms, outpatient care clinics, and many healthcare settings.

They use these techniques when performing surgical procedures, biopsies, dressing wounds, suturing wounds, inserting a urinary catheter, administering injections, and parturition (delivering babies).

Some people mix the words aseptic technique and cleaning technique. Although they are related in which they all aim to keep the hospital and patients clean and protect them from infection, they have some common differences; aseptic techniques are used to eliminate germs that cause diseases, while cleaning techniques are used to decrease the number of microorganisms in the environment.

But all the two techniques are mandatory for any healthcare professional to memorize and put in use.

Mostly, healthcare professionals use cleaning techniques in individuals that are not at high risk of infection. Examples of these cleaning techniques include handwashing, wearing gloves, and always maintaining a clean environment. Cleaning techniques also use the rules of one-touch practice in that they do not allow healthcare professionals to touch key parts of objects like syringe tips inside of sterile dressing, and this rule applies even when they are wearing gloves.

Many medical professionals describe cleaning techniques as a modified way of aseptic techniques that help maintain proper hygiene and a clean environment.

Types of Surgical Aseptic Techniques

Aseptic techniques for the protection of patients are of different types, including:

Barriers: This serves as a protective mechanism between patients and medical professionals. It includes the use of sterile gloves, sterile gowns, sterile masks, sterile drapes, and protective wrappers on the sterilized instruments.

Patients and equipment preparation: this type of aseptic technique ensures that all healthcare professionals and the patients must be prepared before any medical operations occur. These preparations include disinfection of patients' skin using antiseptic wipes, sterilization of equipment before any procedure, storing the sterilized instruments inside plastic wrappers to prevent contamination before use.

Environmental control: The medical procedural area is also called an aseptic field. All medical professionals must ensure that the area where the procedure is going to be carried is clean. This can be done by keeping doors closed and minimizing movement in the aseptic field.

Contacts guidelines: Once the above-mentioned protective mechanisms are achieved, the healthcare professionals must also follow sterile-to-sterile contact guidelines. This contact ensures prohibition between any sterile and non-sterile items contact. Meaning healthcare professionals can only touch sterile items and surfaces and must avoid touching any non-sterile object.

And if any object falls on the ground, the object has to be re-sterilized before using again.

This aseptic technique has a lot of benefits, including:

It entirely helps in protection against infection because when the skin is open, the body is prone to infection, and as known microorganisms are spread everywhere, cuts are always at the risk of infection if care is not taken. The invention of aseptic techniques brought great advancement in the field of medicine and surgery. When a patient needs surgery that has to do with aseptic techniques, they are already prone to infection, so there is a need for the immune system to be at its strongest heal, and there is a great chance of healing fast when the body doesn't have any infection to fight.

CHAPTER 1
Armamentarium (Instrument)

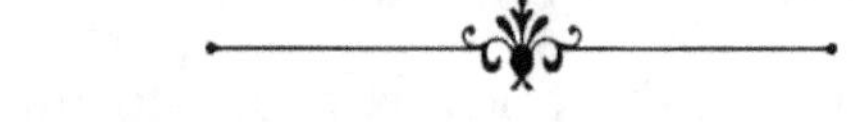

Suture Needles

The use of needles has a long-standing history. It is significantly relevant in today's suture practices. It has been proven as the most cost-effective method compared to mechanical sutures.

Surgical needles are specifically designed and simply used to drive suture materials into the body tissues. They pierce the surface of the skin or other parts and ensure the passage of the materials for the success of the suturing.

There are different types of suture needles, but their usages are based on the location and tissue to be sutured.

Characteristics of the Surgical Needle

1. Flexibility: It should be flexible such that it can bend and not break off.

2. Rigidity: This quality is needed to avoid damage.
3. Sharpness: This is required to ensure ease in penetration into the tissue.
4. Slimness: This is also needed to avoid huge tissue trauma.

Components of a Needle

- End
- Body
- Tip

Needle End

This part is where the suture material is mounted. The end can either be "with an eye" or "without eye/swaged."

Eyed needles	Eyeless or swaged needles
It doesn't have another descriptive name.	They are also known as swaged needles.
It will definitely be threaded with the suture material, primarily through the hole.	Unlike the needle with an eye, here, the suture materials are compressed within the needles.

It inflicts more tissue trauma.	It produces less tissue trauma.
It carries two strands of suture materials through the tissue.	It carries only one strand of suture material through the tissue.
It can be reused.	It should be used just once; hence, infection is of less concern.
It's cost-effective.	

Needle Body

This aspect describes the shape of the needle. Some are straight, curved (1/4, ½, 3/5, and 5/8 of a circle), and half-curved. It should be noted that the curved requires a needle holder and surgical tweezers.

At this juncture, it is important to observe what each is used for.

Straight Needle

It is used for skin closure, which is done by hand; however, it is not always used.

Curved Needle

1/4 of a circle: It is often used in ophthalmic or eye surgery and microsurgery. It is useful for this purpose because of the shallow curvature that makes it easy for convex surfaces.

3/8 of a circle: It is best and commonly used for wounds on the surface level and also large wounds. However, it is not suitable for deep wounds.

1/2 of a circle: It is often used in an enclosed or confined space. Some of those locations in the body are the gastrointestinal tract, respiratory tract, and peritoneum.

5/8 of a circle: It is often used for deep wounds and enclosed or confined spaces. Some of those locations in the body are the gastrointestinal tract, respiratory tract, throat, oral cavity, and urogenital tract.

Half-Curved Needle

This is generally used for laparoscopic surgery.

Needle Tip

This is the part of a needle that has to do with penetration into the body tissues. There is a categorization in this regard, and it's often focused on their cross-sections. That shows the needle's ability to penetrate the tissues.

Needles are classified based on their tips, and this type happens to be the most common such as; reverse cutting, taper cutting, conventional cutting, taper point, etc.

Let's observe them one after the other:

Cutting: Its cross-section is triangle-like, often used for concave surfaces and for tough sclerotic tissue and the sternum.

Reverse Cutting: Unlike the "cutting," its cross-section is in the inverse of the triangle, and it works best on convex surfaces. It is used often for tissues that can tear but are tough, just like the skin.

Spatula: It has a trapezoidal shape, and it's often used for ophthalmic surgeries and microsurgeries.

Round-bodied-tapered: It has a circular shape, and it's often for sutures on the muscle, abdominal viscera, peritoneum, facia, and mucosa.

Blunt round-bodied: This has a circular and round tip. It is used on parenchymatous tissues and ocular muscles.

Now, having seen the meaning of the words suture, suture materials, and suture needle, there is, therefore, a need to understand what instruments are needed to hold the materials and the needle for the success of suturing in any part of the body.

QUICK EXERCISE 1

1. At which year was suturing technique first discovered?

   A. 320BC B. 3000BC C. 6000BC D. 1500BC

2. Who discovered the papyrus of medical knowledge?

   A. Edwith Smith B. Avicenna C. Joseph James D. Muhammad Ali

3. List three characteristics of a surgical needle.

4. List the components of a needle.

5. List the three types of surgical needles.

6. ___________ serves as a protective mechanism between patients and medical professionals; it includes the use of sterile gloves, sterile gowns, sterile

masks, sterile drapes, and protective wrappers on the sterilized instruments.

A. Barrier B. Protection C. Sterile D. Infection

Hand Instruments

Again, these are the instruments required to control and manipulate the needles and suture materials to drive or insert them successfully into the body tissues.

A. Needle Holders: Basically, it is an instrument used to hold the suture needle during suturing. There are two major types:

- Mathieu
- Mayo-Hegar

Characteristics of Needle Holders

- Its handle can be locked.
- It is short-beaked, unlike the artery forceps.
- Cross-hatches and longitudinal grooves are found inside the holder, and it helps to ensure grip on the needle during suturing.
- Its handle can either be long or short. The long is used for deep suturing, while the short handles are used for superficial and delicate suturing.

Handling The Needle Holder

The first rule is that it must be held firmly. However, the knowledge of doing this is germane. Below are the procedures to ensure this:

1. You must insert your thumb and ring finger of your dominant hand in the rings of the needle holder.
2. Your index finger can be used to stabilize the needle holder by putting it on the joints. That would help direct the moves of the needle holder in an attempt to ensure suturing.
3. Now, you are to hold the needle at a perpendicular position to the beak
4. Once this is achieved, there is a ratchet lock on the handle; grasp it to secure it.
5. Afterward, the needle must be removed from the holder by a surgeon.

B. Tissue forceps: The first thing to know about them is that they should be seen as a grasping tool, although they are non-locking. It should be seen as the extension of your thumb.

Purpose of Tissue Forceps

The surgeon or medical professional carrying out the suturing uses this to hold the wound's edges, stabilize tissue, hold the needle, and remove debris in the wound. There are various types of tissue forceps; they are in different sizes but categorized according to the availability of teeth and the type of tissue to be held.

For instance, DeBakey forceps are used for soft tissue and vessels. They are atraumatic.

Toothed Forceps

- Apparently, they have teeth, particularly for dense tissues.
- Those with a single tooth are called "rat teeth," while those in smaller sizes are used for closing wounds. This type is called "Adson."

What should determine whether to use teeth forceps?

- Will it compromise the integrity of the tissues or not?
- What is the amount of tissue to be handled?
- What is the nature of tissue to be handled?

Scissors

Generally, they are specific kinds of scissors used for cutting sutures. Under normal circumstances, this type of scissors should possess a short beak and long handles. The tip of the scissors must always be used to cut and not the flat side of it; doing this ensures the avoidance of trauma done to the tissues.

Types of Scissors

We have Mayo, Metzenbaum, and Iris scissors. Let's observe a brief description of these types of scissors.

- **Mayo scissors:** These types of scissors are of two major types; curved and straight. While the former is used to cut and dissect tissues, the latter is used to cut textiles and sutures.
- **Metzenbaum scissors:** This type is particularly used because of cuts that require precision and for fragile tissues.
- **Iris scissors:** This is primarily used for ophthalmologic operations.

Why the Use of Surgical Instruments?

This is a general question that is often asked by aspiring medical personnel.

To be a successful surgeon, mastering the surgical instrument is important. The names and use of each surgical instrument will be given later. This chapter comprises why surgical instruments are important in the act of surgery and suturing.

Surgical instruments are tools or equipment that are specifically used to perform a surgery or operation. Nowadays, many surgical instruments have been invented. While some are specially designed for a type of surgery, others are designed for a particular procedure. Most of the surgical instruments follow certain patterns. For example, a tracheotome is a tool used to perform a tracheotomy. These surgical instruments are mostly made from stainless steel, metals, and alloys like Titanium and Vitallium. A package of surgical instruments consists of specific tools designated for a particular surgery. The purpose of using a surgical instrument, especially in suturing, is to avoid infection, help to stop bleeding, and to provide a visually pleasing scar rather than a grotesque tissue mass. It is also essential to consider the suturing materials when performing an operation. It is always easy to select the right suturing instrument by considering the location and nature of a wound. Another purpose of using surgical instruments is to minimize skin tension.

Surgical Blades

For every successful surgery, there is a need for perfect surgical blades, especially in suturing.

Most medical students are known to have that anxiety when they first visit a suturing room because the theatre room is a place with many strict rules and regulations. But mastering the instruments that are going to be used for an operation tends to help in reducing the tension, their names, and the purpose of each. While other instruments can be reused after sterilization, some, like syringes, can only be used once.

In this book, everything is simplified. Below is a list and detailed explanation of types of surgical blades, their sizes, and their uses.

Scalpel

This is one of the oldest and still-in-use surgical instruments known in every hospital facility. It has many purposes, which will be detailed later. It is also a tool with a Bard-Parker Handle.

Recently, Alloys like stainless steel have been used in manufacturing the scalpel, which is reusable and has high resistance to corrosion.

Types of Blades

There are different types of blades that are divided based on the type of surgery and the type of incision. These blades have different sizes and shapes and are labeled using numbers. They also have compatible handles, which are also numbered according to their respective sizes.

Handle No. 3

It is the most common handle used for incision. Its compatible blades are Blade No. 10, 11, 12, and 15. It has two subtypes which are 3G and 3L.

Handle No. 4

This is the same as handle No. 3 but with a larger till to accommodate larger blades. It is compatible with blades No. 20, 21, 22, 23, and 26. It has two subtypes, which are 4G and 4L.

Handle No. 7

This is a tall and slender handle used in making incisions in tight and deep body areas. It is compatible with blades No. 10, 11, 12, and 15.

Blades And Their Descriptions

1. Blade No. 10: This is a blade used in making skin incisions. It has a curved belly which is a sharp edge.

2. Blade No. 11: It is a straight angle edge with a pointed end. It is used for making stabs in cases where a drain needs to be inserted.

3. Blade No. 12: This s a crescent-shaped blade with the inner crescent curvature being the sharp edge. It is used for the removal of sutures and cleft palate and parotid surgeries.

4. Blade No. 15: The cutting edge of this blade is small. It is similar to blade No. 10, but it is shorter. It is used for making short and precise incisions.

5. Blade No. 20: This is similar to blade No. 10, but it is bigger. It is a curved belly blade with the curved side being the sharp edge. It is used in making skin incisions.

6. Blade No. 21: It is similar to blade No. 10 but larger than blade No. 20. It is a curved belly blade with the curved part as the edge. It is used for making skin incisions.

7. Blade No. 22: It is similar to blade No. 10 but larger than blade no.21, having a curved belly with the curved side as the sharp side. It is used in making skin incisions.

8. Blade No. 23: It is a leaf-shaped blade. It also has a curved cutting edge. It is used for making long incisions.

9. Blade No. 26: This blade has a straight cutting edge.

How To Use The Scalpel

For every surgery to be carried out successfully, there has to be an incision; it is one of the most important and first acts done. The scalpel is used in making these incisions. In the Operating Theater, the scalpel is one of the most important instruments used, and it can be held in different ways based on the type of incision that needs to be done.

1. **Palmer Grip:** This is a grip is used when making incisions on tough tissues. The handle is held in between the 5th, middle and ring finger, and placing the index finger over the border of the handle.

2. **Pencil Grip:** This type of grip is done just as holding a pencil. This type of grip is used in making small and precise cuts with the handle

placed over the palm. The movement in this grip is from the finger to make fine cuts.

3. **Finger-Tip Grip:** It is the modified palmer grip used in making longer incisions, usually on the skin

4. **Stab Grip:** It is a modified palmer grip with the scalpel held at 90° to the skin's surface. It is used during laparoscopic surgeries.

QUICK EXERCISE 2

1. _____________ is a blade use in making skin incision. It has a curved belly which is a sharp edge.

   A. Blade No. 10 B. Blade No. 9 C. Blade No. 12 D. Blade No. 14

2. _____________ is the type of grip used in making small and precise cuts with the handle placed over the palm

   A. Pencil grip B. Cleaner grip C. Stab grip D. Finger-tip grip

3. _____________ is used for skin closure which is done by hand.

   A. Straight needle B. Curved needle C. Bend needle D. Hand needle

4. List the three types of surgical scissors.

CHAPTER 2
Purpose and Basic Principles of Suturing

Alien, a twenty-two-year-old university student, had an accident yesterday morning and had a deep cut around her leg which she kept to herself and decided to clean up with tap water since she was getting tired by the moment. No one was around to take her to the PHC around her house, which was always filled with people. Having lost so much blood and getting tired by each passing minute, she reached for her purse and snapped for pain-relieving drugs and antibiotics. She took two pills, reached for a bandage with plaster, and used it to cover it up, hoping that the blood clot would close up the cut and she would get fine. It was around 9:00 pm. Having managed to endure the pain, her sleeping gate was left open as her cries for help filtered the neighborhood. The leg, while infected, had also retained fluid and couldn't be lifted from one area to the other. Her shout got her neighbor, who was now back from work. Her neighbor rushed to help her to the hospital as she couldn't relate to her plight, but it was obvious that something was wrong with her. She was in pain. As one who has the knowledge of suturing, proffer solution as to what she should have done?

Consider another case scenario, Becca, a 20-year-old secondary school student, was at work in her mother's shop trying to separate wrongly joined fabrics unknown to her that her forefinger was way too close to the razor blade, she was trying to cut the fabrics unknown to her that her fingers were present and as such, she sustained a minor cut while she unconsciously placed the finger in her mouth and later wrapped it with a piece of cloth to reduce bleeding. What should she have done to her sustained injury?

These and many more are day-to-day life cycles that happen around us, when and where to use suture in relation to cuts or lacerations, wounds; wounds that have an increased risk of infection, facial wounds, deep wounds that goes down to the fat, muscle, bone or other deep structures, wounds that continue to bleed after 15 minutes of direct pressure, etc. become a question for the professional in training to find out while having the knowledge of the purpose of suturing which this chapter will cover extensively.

Why Suturing?

While the term is very common, well expatiated in the first chapter, thinking everyone knows the nitty-gritty of what it entails and reasons for going through the process of suturing is one reason this book should not have come into existence at all. A book at its best should do what a book does, inform the audience or the reader on how best or close to best, to approach matters as relating to what is explained. With this information, it is important to know how and where suturing is needed, when to use it to support and strengthen wounds until healing, reduce dead space, approximate skin edges, reduce scarring, and reduce the risk of bleeding and infection. That, however, portrays that for the objectives of suturing to be achieved, indications and contra-indications, location, and the type of wounds or cuts should be considered. While Alien and Becca's case are both wounds, one needs to be sutured as a result of the type of wound and perhaps the location, while the other needs to be treated with first aid, and that will be all to ensure healing. This also implies that the risk of infection of an open wound increases the longer the wound remains open, and wound that may require closure should be stitched, closed, or stapled. Not assuming that you know whose case needs suturing, but can you guess whose? Yes, you are right. It is Alien's case.

Objectives, Indications and Contraindications of Suturing

This section has only one main use to do justice to the objectives and indications of suturing while explaining the basic principles that should guide the placement of any type of suture. Having discussed what a suture is and what a suture material is made up of, it's important to look at the objectivity of stitching a wound:

Objectives Of Suturing

In the wound healing process or closure of cutaneous wounds, the technique has remained the same, the materials and aspects of the technique have changed spontaneously with time, and the primary reason sometimes referred to as the "objective of suturing," has simply not deviated from its scope, these include:

- To have two separated edges of a wound brought back together so they can remain in contact as in their natural state before the accident to facilitate cell repair, cell regeneration, and cell growth while preventing the excessive growth of new tissues, which may create disfiguration, imbalance to the homeostatic state of the body system and yet not heal if left to stay without suturing.

- To enhance wound healing by providing tensile strength until the natural healing process of the body starts to incorporate the needed tensile strength (production of collagen fibers) between the newly opposed edges.

- To exclude dead spaces which when open between layers of wounds, could cause further decomposition and enhance the incidence of infection.

- To reduce blood loss and further bleeding, which flows as a result of tissue damage, if further bleeding is not controlled, loss of blood could lead to a shortage of blood while coma sets in, death may not be far off within a short period.

- To reduce infestation of infectious agents. When wounds are formed, the body's immune system is compromised while its inner layer, which has been kept in sterile form, is abridged. This, in a way, causes the balance to shift the sterility of the membranes unsterile and the introduction of microbes. This is one of the reasons the wound has to be dressed and closed.

Indications For Securing Sutures

- To ensure tissue wounds get healed and tissues get back to their natural state unless in a contraindicated state in which wounds are less severe, such as in the case of abrasion. It can be taken care of by keeping it open yet treated.

- In cases where the skin cut creates a flap of tissues, which has to be secured back at their recipient site, the suture is needed to bridge the gap.

- To restore certain congenital conditions (defects) such as craniosynostosis, scaphocephaly needs surgical attention and suturing.

- To network and transfix broken blood vessels in order to achieve balance and homeostasis in the human system.

- To restore broken blood vessels together in order to channel the blood flow to a new anatomical site.

- To restore separated nerves and tendons to their natural state.

- To secure drains which include tracheostomy, nasogastric, and gastronomy tubes and prevent them from interfering with the body's fluids.

- To retract tissues so as to ameliorate access and visibility.

- To help secure pen flaps of tissue over a bone.

Contraindications For Suturing

When the bruise, wound, or cut is superficial, there would be no reason to suture as it will go through natural healing without a suture. Remember, such an example was made available; minor cuts, wounds, bruises on curved surfaces of the body, such as the nasal alar crease and preauricular sulcus, are better allowed to get healed naturally if not severe. Wounds that are kept closed to microbes are not to be sutured, and those opened to microbes and not treated before suturing are not to be treated lest there is a multiplication of infectious agents within. This can only be done if microbes have been controlled and overlying delicate soft tissues are not to be sutured tightly. Sutures ensure that tissues are held firmly, not too tight, lest they cause trauma to the affected skin, ischemia, and death of the tissue while eventually tearing up cannot be saved. All these, put together, are what is referred to as contraindication of suturing. In other words, the type of wounds or wound's location that opposes the indication of suturing.

Basic Principles of Suturing

Considering that there are different principles on suturing, certain basic principles cannot be omitted while securing a suture. While learning the art of suturing as a beginner or student, a lot of observation has to be made to prevent causing more harm than good before practice is done. The procedural principles are to be closely followed. Sooner than you know, with practice and observation, it becomes well known as the back of your palm.

Principles of Using an Armamentarium

- Before suturing, keep in mind that you are to hold the needle and suture materials in the best position, as shown below, as it is mandatorily important.

- Have the needle holder placed in your dominant hand so that you don't have it screwed up, with the positions between your thumb and ring finger.

- Position the needle in the jaws of the needle holder at 90^0 to it both vertically and horizontally.

- Have the needle held at a point that its holder is at a point that it lies in the holder One-third in length to the distance from the eye of the needle and two-thirds from the tip.

- Position the tissue forceps to be held in your non-dominant hand, grasping as though you were using a pen.

Many terms will still be laid out, but let us be introduced to what it means to have a bite during suturing as likened to the common bite. It is done just once and could be done on any material of concern.

A **Bite** is a process of thrusting the needle into the tissue and withdrawing it to secure part of the open wound or cut, to have this done in the right way so as to prevent further damage of the tissue. These basic principles of a bite should be followed:

- Utilize the tissue forceps to pick up the suturing process in stages from the edge of the wound and backtrack or revert it gently. Doing this will help you see and observe how the needle leaves from the opposite side.

- Utilize the needle to penetrate the tissue on one side of the wound while measuring the ideal distance before inserting it into neighboring tissue as 5 mm from the edge of the wound. While the word "utilize" has been used on different occasions, it is of worthy note to know that your needle is a tool in your hands, and mastering it helps you produce better craft and, in this case, not anything but on humans.

- Remember, the needle must penetrate the tissue at right angles to the surface of the wound. This allows it to pierce through the wound better without causing atraumatic fashion.

- Notice the point of entrance of the needle; ensure you push the needle further into the tissue. While doing that, try pushing it following the natural curvatures of the needle; this is less traumatic and provides the least resistance from the tissue.

- Observe as the needle exits on the inner side of the tissue while the needle holder is released from entering the end of the needle while using it to hold the emerging end of the needle.

- Pull the needle with the suture material intact out of the inner wound edge while following the natural needle curvature.

- Remember, the bite must be taken through the neighboring (2nd) wound edge. Take the bite at the inner edge of the second side (this may vary according to the technique chosen) (techniques to be discussed soon).

- The same principle given previously for entering and exiting the second wound edge should be followed.

- The distance of the bites taken on both sides should be equal to prevent loosening back, tissue damage, or unequal suturing. Therefore, it's best if the first bite taken was 5 mm from the wound edge. The second bite must also have an exit that is 5 mm from the edge to ensure uniformity and precision. Resist the temptation of taking both bites simultaneously.

- Taking each bite separately gives you time to ensure the needed patience takes its due and full course while also saving your time and incorporating accuracy in your suture. Similarly, the depth of the bite should not stay unequal through the region to be sutured except in cases that have to do with the dermal-subdermal suture technique.

- How you position a suture is also a concern in ensuring a smooth process. While sutures are done to get tissue flaps together, they are conducted to ensure adequate access while limiting unnecessary tension. Caution is to be observed in every part of the tissue to be sutured. For instance, the edge sutured away from you, and the other edge sutured towards you or from your dominant side to non-dominant side. However, certain rules have proven best over time when considering different tissues. For instance, fixed and moveable tissues always suture from moveable tissues to fixed tissues to ensure firmness and quick healing.

- When there is a non-uniformity of thickness in what is to be sutured, always suture from thinner tissues to thicker tissues and also consider depths. Suturing should be done from deeper tissues to more superficial tissues.

The general rules of suturing, which may also be known as stitching rules, are as follows:

- It must not be too close to the end of the margin of the wound.
- Place the suture at the same distance.
- Knots, placed out of the wound line to prevent it from loosening up or uneven suturing.
- Stitches should be done cleanly with evenness and accuracy, not trial and error methods that could cause tissue trauma. Over-turning the

edges of the wound should be avoided except in purse-string ligature.

Suturing is a form of surgical operation and can be classified according to layers, one layer if we only approximate one of the tissues; two or more layers can be considered, according to depth, one or two rarely more lines and according to the length which could be interrupted or continues suture lines of the skin. These different types of Sutures are outlined below:

- **Simple Interrupted Sutures:** This is the most often used, adaptable, and simplest suture, as its name implies in cutaneous surgery. The needle is inserted perpendicular to the epidermis to place this suture. Traverse the epidermis as well as the entire thickness of the dermis before exiting perpendicular to the epidermis with the epidermis on the wound's opposing side while the stitch is on both sides. In terms of depth and width, it is symmetrically situated. The suture should, in general, have a flask-like appearance configuration. For instance, the stitch should be broader at the base (dermal side) than at the top (Subcutaneous side). The epidermis, the outermost layer of the skin (epidermal side), should have the stitch encircling its larger area of tissue at one time because the tissue is compressed at its base rather than its apex while the tissue is forced upward. This encourages wound edges to evert. This strategy lowers the chances of forming a bond. As the wound heals, the scar becomes depressed.

As of the image below:

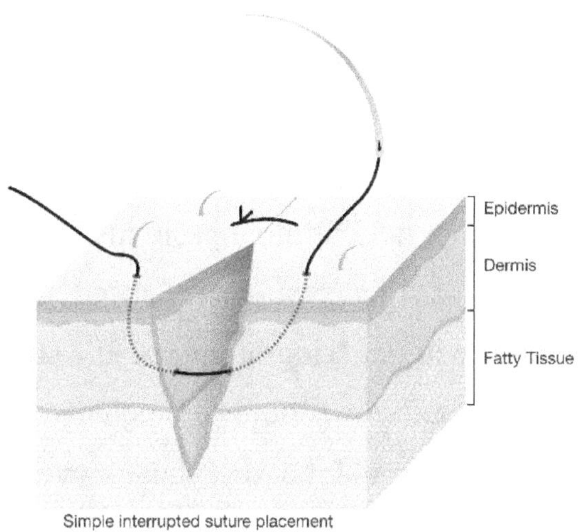

Simple interrupted suture placement

To avoid the potential of mismatched wound-edge heights, tissue bites should not be crowded but be evenly spaced, as discussed above, and it is to be ensured that the wound edges meet at the same level (stepping). However, when the distance of the needle insertion site from the wound edge and that of the needle exit site are varied from the wound edge, the bite's depth corresponds to the size of the bite taken from the two sides of the wound's size and can be deliberately altered. Asymmetry in edge thickness or height can be corrected by using different-sized needle bites on each side of the incision. Small bites can be utilized to close wound edges nearby. To relieve wound tension, large bites might be employed. To ensure exact wound approximation while avoiding tissue strangulation, proper tension is essential.

- **Simple Running Sutures:** This consists of a series of simple uninterrupted sutures that run in a continuous pattern. The suture is started by tying but not cutting a basic interrupted stitch. A series of simple sutures are inserted one after the other without tying or cutting the suture material pass. Sutures should be equally spaced, and tension should be distributed evenly over the length of the suture. Line of suture, the knot is tied between the suture material's tail end and the point where it departs the body's wound as well as the last suture loop.

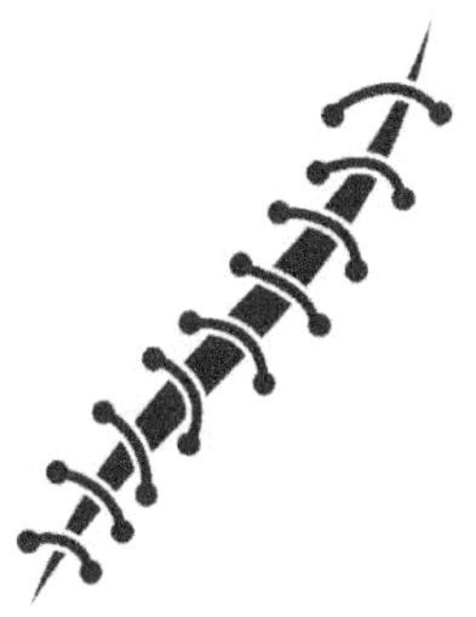

- **Running Locked Suture:** It is possible to have a suture locked or unlocked and still be termed as a basic running suture. A running locked suture's first knot is known as it is locked by passing the needle through the loop before it as the stitch is made. The final appearance of this running locked suture line, a kind of suture, is known as baseball stitch.

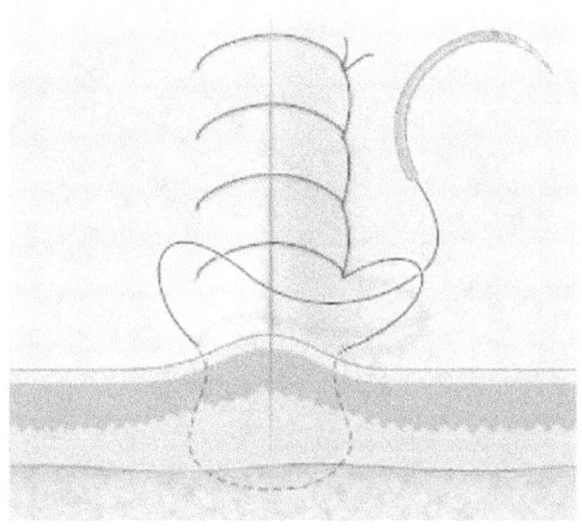

- **Vertical Mattress Suture:** This version of the simple interrupted suture is one of the best suturing of wounds to ensure eversion of wounds and eliminate significant wound tension while it consists of a wide, deep interrupted stitch and a second more superficial interrupted stitch placed closer to the wound edge and in the opposite direction, while in accordance to the amount of stress on the wound, the width of the stitch should be raised. This is to show that the broader the stitch, the higher the tension. This should no longer be new to you, as it has been discussed during the principles of stitching.

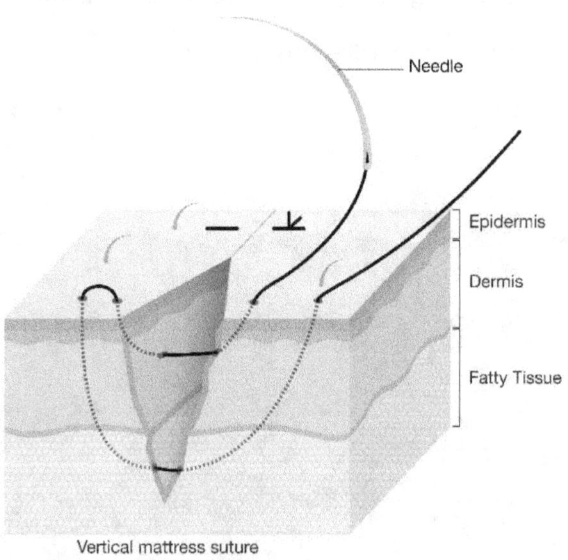

Vertical mattress suture

- **Half–Buried Vertical Mattress Suture:** The half-buried vertical mattress suture is a variation on the vertical mattress suture that annuls two of the four points resulting in less scarring. The needle used to penetrate the skin goes into the deep part of the dermis on the side of the wound, takes a bite in the deep part of the dermis without exiting the skin then, crosses back to the first side of the wound, and leaves the skin just as in the case of the vertical mattress suture. Therefore, only a side of the wound is useful for both entry and exit.

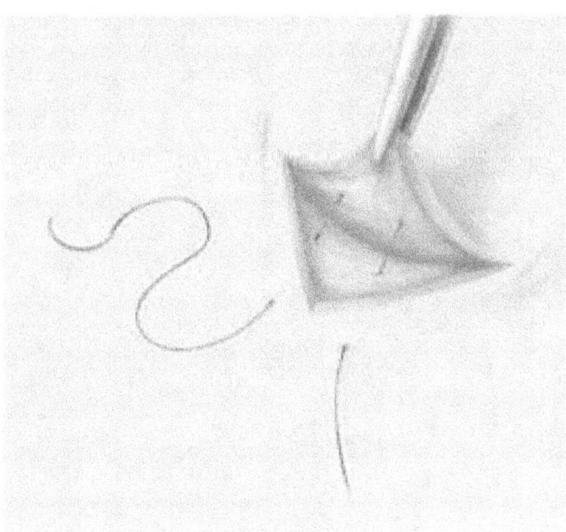

Figure 3. Half-buried mattress sutures.

- **Horizontal Mattress Suture:** In this suture, the skin is entered by having the needle penetrate 5 mm to 1 cm from the wound edge. The suture is passed deep to the opposite side of the suture line as it leaves the skin the same distance from the wound edge (just like a deep, simple interrupted stitch). The needle reenters the skin on the same side of the suture line 5 mm to about 1 cm lateral of the exit point. The stitch is passed deep to the other side of the wound, where it leaves the skin, and the knot is tied. It is then put in place, helping in minimizing wound tension, closing the dead space, and facilitating wound edge eversion.

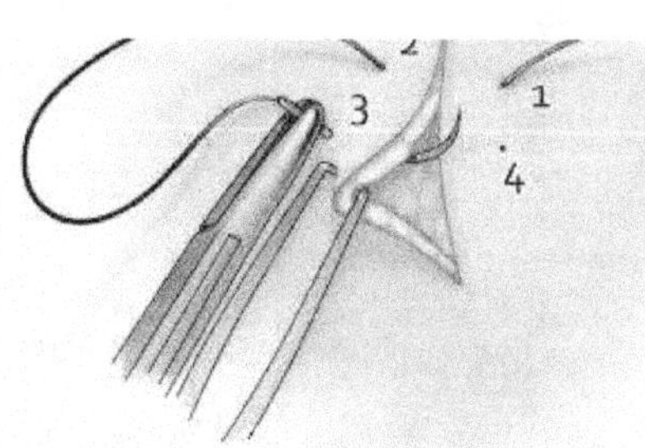

B. Continuous

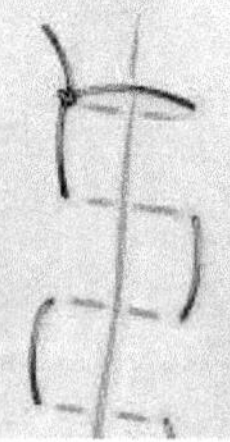

Process Of Wound Healing

It is generally known that the skin is the largest organ in the body, and one of the many important functions of the skin is to serve as a cover to the body and also a barrier to protect the body against any infection.

The skin has three layers.

> ➢ The epidermis which is the outermost layer
> ➢ The dermis, which is the middle layer
> ➢ The Hypodermis is the innermost layer.

When a wound happens, it occurs due to a breakdown of the integrity of the epidermal layer of the skin. Let us quickly examine the types of wounds that we have:

1. Abrasions: This is the type of wound that occurs as a result of brushing off part of the body against a blunt or rough surface. Minimal bleeding usually occurs; the dermis is unaffected and does not require suturing as in bruising of the calf following brushing against the floor

2. Lacerations: This type of wound occurs as a result of sharp objects tearing, slicing, or cutting through the skin. It may affect the epidermis alone or the

three skin layers and even cut through the blood vessels. A lacerated wound may be clean as in a Surgical incision or haggard as in a glass. The use of sutures is evident in deep lacerations

3. Punctures: This type of wound results from pointed objects projected at a very high degree such that penetration occurs. Punctures are to be carefully examined in that they might have caused internal bleeding. A punctured wound can be from Gunshot, knife stab, glass stab, or any sharp object causing penetration.

4. Exploration of the wound is important, especially when internal bleeding occurs, and it usually involves suturing.

5. Avulsions: This is a very extensive wound characterized by body tissues torn away from the rest of the body. It is life-threatening and requires a series of interventions like skin grafting, cosmetic surgery, etc. It is usually caused by road traffic accidents or explosions.

Although wound healing might look complex and complicated, it's easy, especially when reading this book.

Wound healing generally means healing of the skin after an injury. The body is a complex system. The changes that occur during a wound explain how the body works together with all the systems and tissues in repairing and replacing damaged cells and tissues. But the ultimate question remains: how does the body heal?

Types Of Wound Healing

Wound healing is generally classified into two;

- Primary wound healing
- Secondary wound healing

Primary wound healing: This non-complicated healing occurs in a non-infected or small wound, e.g., surgical wound.

Secondary wound healing: This is a complicated wound healing that occurs due to infection, e.g., immune system dysfunction.

Wound healing is often easier in children than in adults. This is because children's bodies and immune systems are not as complicated as that of adults.

When an injury occurs, the body immediately stands in motion to coordinate a series of events called a cascade of healing to repair the injured tissues. In adults, this cascade of healing is divided into four phases:

- ✓ Hemostasis Phase
- ✓ Inflammatory Phase
- ✓ Proliferative Phase
- ✓ Maturation Phase

Let us have them explained in detail below

Hemostasis Phase

The word hemostasis refers to the arrest or stoppage of bleeding.

Hemostasis is the body occurs in three stages.

1. **Vascular-Constriction:** When an injury occurs, the blood vessels, arteries, and arterioles constrict in other to stop the bleeding; this is a local phenomenon. When blood vessels are cut due to injury, the body's endothelial gets damaged, and collagen gets exposed. Platelet adheres to the exposed collagen and gets activated. The platelet that got activated secretes some neurotransmitters like serotonin which causes constriction of blood vessels.

2. **Platelet Plug Formation:** In this stage, the platelet adheres to the collagen of the ruptured blood vessels and secrete some substances like adenosine diphosphate (ADP) and thromboxane A2; these two substances help to attract more and more platelet then activate them. These platelets that get activated aggregate and form a temporary loose platelet Plug. This loose platelet Plug temporarily closes the ruptured blood vessels.

3. **Coagulation of Blood:** In this stage, fibrinogen is converted to fibrin. The fibrin gets attached to that loose platelet plugin stage two and completely blocks the blood vessels, blocking further blood loss.

Inflammatory Phase

The second phase of wound healing is the inflammatory phase. This occurs immediately after the injury occurs. The injured blood vessels release transudate, a mixture of water, salts, and protein, which causes localized swelling. But inflammation has the benefit of controlling bleeding and the spread of infection. The fluid engorgement permits healing and repairing cells to move to the site of injury. During this phase, damaged cells, pathogens, and bacteria are removed from the injury site. White blood cells, known as the first line of defense in the body, growth factors, nutrients, and enzymes form the swelling, heat, and pain that are commonly seen during this phase of wound healing. Inflammation is naturally part of wound healing. But it can become a problem when it becomes prolonged or extensive.

Proliferative Phase

This stage occurs when the wound is rebuilt with new tissue formed by collagen and extracellular matrix.

The process that occurs in this phase is that as new tissues are built, the wound contracts. For the granulation tissue to be healthy with a maximum supply of oxygen and nutrients, a new arrangement of blood vessels has to be built. The wound contracts due to myofibroblasts, which causes the gripping of the wound edges by pulling them together using a mechanism that looks like a smooth muscle cells mechanism. The granulation tissue of the healing process is pink or red, and the texture is uneven, and it's known that granulation tissues do not bleed easily. When there is the appearance of dark granulation tissue, it indicates the presence of infection, ischemia, or poor perfusion. Finally, the epithelial cells resurface the injury. This epithelialization occurs faster when wounds are kept moist and hydrated. But when occlusive or semi-occlusive dressings are applied within 48 hours after the injury. They help in maintaining correct tissue humidity and optimizing epithelialization.

Maturation Phase

This stage is also called the remodeling stage and is the last stage of the healing process.

In this phase, collagen is remodeled from type III to type I, and the wound then closes fully. Apoptosis or programmed cell death helps in removing the cells that were used for the repairing of the damaged tissues. Now the collagen is laid down during the proliferative stage, it is then disorganized, and the wound becomes thick. The collagen exposed during the hemostasis state became remodeled into a more organized structure along the lines of stress. It then increases the tensile strength of the healing tissues. Fibroblast then secretes the enzyme matrix metalloproteinases, which facilitate remodeling of the type III collagen to type I collagen.

This remodeling process begins about 21 days after an injury and can continue for a year or more.

When there is any disruption in the process of wound healing, it can lead to excessive wound healing or chronic wound formation. This excessive wound healing occurs when the pathogenesis of the excessive wound healing is not fully understood, and it's an abnormal wound healing that results in continuous localized inflammation. In contrast, chronic wound formation is a wound that fails to heal for a period of 4 weeks. This might occur due to age, weak immune system, malnutrition, insufficient oxygen supply, diseases, smoking, radiation, and many other factors.

Other complications associated with wound healing include:

Formation of deficient scar, exuberant granulation, deficient contraction, or excessive contractions, especially in burns.

Factors That Can Affect Wound Healing

A lot of factors can affect wound healing, whether the wound is due to injury or surgery; they include:

Age of the patient: Nany healing capacities are associated with age, especially due to some physical changes that occur with advanced age. Studies have shown that people who are 60 above have poor wound healing than those below the age of 60. This happens as a result of a decrease in the body's inflammatory response. Some changes occur visibly in the skin, like age spots and dry skin, which occur due to a reduction in the function of sebaceous glands. There is also a decrease in collagen synthesis, which causes slower scar formation in the process of healing.

The type of wound: The type of wound also affects the healing process because it's obvious that large wounds take more time to heal than small wounds, and the shape of a wound also plays a role in determining the rate of healing. Also, linear wounds always heal faster than rectangular wounds, while circular wounds are the slowest to heal. However, wound healing tends to be slower when there is the presence of necrotic tissue, dedication, and foreign bodies.

Infection: The presence of wounds gives a chance for harmful substances like bacteria, viruses, or fungus to enter. But amazingly, white blood cells being the body's protective soldiers, eliminate the unwanted substances along with some components of the immune system. To treat this infection, sometimes, the use of antibiotics is sufficient.

Chronic disease: People suffering from underlined health issues like diabetes tend to have a low healing mechanism. For a wound to heal, it requires an adequate blood flow.

Poor nutrition: Poor nutrition can cause slowing of wound healing. The infection causes an increase in protein and calories needed in the body. Normally, wounds exude a large number of proteins daily, so when there is an insufficiency of nutrients, the body tends to break down protein for energy resulting in further depletion in the ability of the body to heal.

Dehydration: When there is a decrease in the water supply to the body, which results in loss of moisture at the wound surface and a decrease in blood oxygenation, this can slow down the healing process. A properly hydrated patient will have clear and odorless urine.

Decrease Blood Circulation: The properties necessary for wound healing are transported in the blood, so when there is a decrease in blood circulation, automatically, there will be a delay in the healing process.

Edema: When edema becomes excessive, it leads to an increase in pressure in blood vessels, which results in decreased blood circulation to the site of injury.

Continuous Trauma: Re-injury of the infected site or pressure against the site of infection can cause a delay in the healing process.

The Behavior of Patients: Some patients contribute to the slow healing process, especially through some lifestyle behaviors like smoking, inadequate sleep, inadequate wound dressing procedure, and not keeping the wound moist.

Process Of Fracture Healing

The fracture healing process might look complex, but it's actually easy. One amazing thing about bone healing is a bone is among the tissues that can heal without forming a scar.

Types Of Fracture Healing

Fracture healing is classified into two categories:

- Direct or primary fracture healing
- Indirect or secondary fracture healing

Direct or primary fracture healing occurs when the bones are fixed with compression, and there is no formation of callus. Osteoclast and osteoblast activities join the bony ends.

Generally, indirect healing is common than direct healing because it involves endochondral and intramembranous bone healing. And also, there is no need for an anatomical reduction. Rather, a small amount of motion and weight-bearing at the site of the fracture causes the formation of callus, leading to the formation of secondary bone. Note that too much weight on site of injury or unnecessary movement can cause a delay in the process of healing.

Phases of indirect healing;

Below are phases or stages of indirect healing

Acute inflammatory response: This is an important stage for healing to occur; it's a peak that occurs within 24hrs to 7days. In this stage, a hematoma is formed immediately after the injury. Also, this comprises cells from peripheral and intramedullary blood and bone marrow cells. Hematoma coagulation around the fracture ends and within the medulla due to the inflammatory response. Necrosis factors are also released to improve the process of healing and blood vessel growth.

Recruitment of mesenchymal **stem cells:** Without proper recruitment of mesenchymal stem cells, bones fail to regenerate, leading to a slower fracture healing process.

Generation of cartilaginous and periosteal bony callus: Fibrin-rich granulation tissue forms after the hematoma has been formed. Also, between the fracture ends and beyond the periosteal site of the tissues, there is the formation of endochondral that is less stable and allows the cartilaginous tissue to form the soft callus simultaneously, giving the fracture additional stability.

Revascularization and neoangiogenesis: For a bone to repair properly, there is a need for an adequate blood supply. For this, chondrocytes apoptosis and cartilaginous degradation are important to ensure the removal of extracellular matrix and movement of blood vessels to the repair site.

Mineralization and resorption of the cartilaginous callus: For bone regeneration to continue, the primary soft cartilaginous callus has to be resorbed and replaced by the hard-cartilaginous callus.

Bone remodeling: Although the hard callus might look rigid and stable, that does not mean the site of fracture has fully restored all the properties of normal bone, and for that, a second restorative stage is essential. In this stage, remodeling of the hard callus into a patellar bone structure attached with a central medullary cavity occurs.

When lamellar bone is deposited by osteoblast and callus is resorbed by osteoclasts, this determines the occurrence of remodeling. It also results from the production of electrical polarity and when pressure is applied in a crystalline environment.

Electropositive convex and electronegative concave are created when axial loading of long bone occurs, activating osteoclast and osteoblast activities. Due to this, lamellar bone structure slowly replaces the external callus. Simultaneously, remodeling of the internal callus occurs, which recreates a medulla cavity that resembles diaphyseal bone.

For bone remodeling to occur successfully, there is a need for an adequate supply of blood and an increase in mechanical stability so as to avoid any complications.

Direct Fracture Healing

In this stage, there is a need for a decrease in fracture ends and without the formation of any gap or stable fixation. This phase does not occur naturally but with open reduction and internal fixation surgery. Direct bone healing occurs by directly remodeling the lamellar bone, Haversian canals, and the blood vessels. And the process normally takes months to years.

Direct fracture healing occurs through the following processes:

Contact healing and gap healing. The two processes comprise an attempt to recreate the lamellar bone structure. Also, for direct healing to occur, it requires compression of the fracture ends and rigid fixation to reduce the interfragmentary strain.

Contact Healing

This is another form of bone healing, where the fracture can unite when the gap between each bone end is Less than 0.01 mm, and the interfragmentary strain is below 2%. When this happens, cones are cut at the end of the osteons by the fracture site. And the tip of the cut cones comprises of osteoclasts. These tips cross the fracture line and generate a cavity. The cavity will then be tiller by bone that was produced by the osteoblast. This leads to the union of the bones simultaneously restoring the Haversian systems, which were formed by the axial direction. This Haversian allows blood vessels that are carrying osteoblast to enter the affected area. Then the osteons that bridge slowly mature into lamellar bones, which leads to fracture healing without a periosteal callus formation.

Gap Healing

This is a unique form of fracture healing in which bony union and Haversian remodeling forms do not occur at once. And for this process to happen, the gap between the bone must be below 8.00 mm to 1 mm. Lamellar bone filler is the fracture site that runs perpendicular to the long axis and needs secondary osteons formation. Longitudinal revascularized osteons slowly replace the primary bone structure that carries osteoprogenitor cells which differentiate into osteoblast. The osteoblast further produces lamellar bones on each surface of the gap. This lamellar bone is laid perpendicular to the long axis, meaning it is not strong. It takes about 3-4 weeks for this process to occur. After this process, the secondary remodeling phase occurs, which resembles the cascade with cutting cones in the contact healing explained above.

Factors Affecting Fracture Healing

A lot of factors affect fracture healing which results in slow healing. These factors are detailed below:

<u>Blood Supply</u>: When there is an inadequate supply of blood in the blood, it greatly affects the process of fracture healing and all kinds of healing processes in the body.

<u>Soft Tissue Injury</u>: A strain or sprain is a common tissue injury that occurs in the body when there is damage in muscles, ligaments, and tendons in the body. This mechanism is termed soft tissue injury, and it affects the process of fracture healing. It can also occur due to continuous use of a particular body part, especially the injury site.

<u>Age</u>: Age greatly affects the process of fracture healing; people of older age tend to heal slower than people of younger age.

<u>Infection</u>: The occurrence of infection affects fracture healing. Some of the cases may lead to severe damage to the patient's body.

<u>Anemia or hypoxia</u>: Anemia is the decrease in the production of red blood cells, while hypoxia is the

decrease in the availability of oxygen in the tissues; when these two occur, the healing rate tends to be slower than normal.

<u>Excessive compression:</u> Normally, compression of fractures can cause breakage of bone, talk less of when it is done in excess; this can highly slow the rate of bone healing and sometimes cause severe damage to the site of injury.

<u>Excessive movement:</u> Staying in one place and avoiding excessive movement increases the rate of healing, while excessive movement slows fracture healing.

<u>Gap:</u> Excess gap between bones also causes slow healing of fractures.

<u>Nutrition:</u> Poor hygiene and inadequate supply of nutrients required for the body cause slow healing of fractures.

<u>Drugs:</u> Drugs like cytotoxic antineoplastic and immunosuppressive agents, corticosteroids, nonsteroidal anti-inflammatory drugs, and anticoagulants cause slow healing of not only fractures but in wounds entirely in the body.

QUICK EXERCISE 3

1. _____________ excludes dead spaces which, when opened between layers of wound, could cause further decomposition and enhance the incidence of infection.

   A. Suturing B. Bone healing c. Bone remodeling D. Wound dehiscence

2. Fracture healing is classified into ________ categories?

   A. 4 B. 3 C. 2 D. 1

3. _____________ is the process of thrusting the needle into the tissue and withdrawing it to secure part of the open wound or cut, to have this done in the right way so as to prevent further damage of the tissue.

   A. Suture B. Bone repair C. Bite D. Techniques

4. ___________ is a variation on the vertical mattress suture that eliminates two of the four entry points resulting in less scarring.

5. Half-buried vertical mattress suture B. Complete-buried vertical mattress suture C. Partially-buried vertical mattress suture D. Incomplete-buried vertical mattress suture.

6. When a wound happens, it occurs as a result of ___________ of the integrity of the epidermal layer of the skin.

   A. Breakdown B. Remodeling C. Correction D. Cutting

7. ___________ is not among the factors that can affect wound healing.

   A. Age B. Infection C. Food D. Edema

CHAPTER 3
Surgical Knots

In the suture technique, very fundamental are the surgical knots. These surgical knots are used in every suture technique and specifically at the end of the suture. The surgical knots are used to secure the suture in place to avoid any distortion of the work already concluded. They are very fundamental and cannot be overemphasized. The knot is described by several physicians as the "weakest" link. The probity or wholeness of an entire suture is greatly dependent on the integrity of the surgical knot. This means that the beauty and effectiveness of an entire suture, after all has been said and done, is dependent on the surgical knot. The need for a secure knot is that if this knot is not secure, it can lead to the occurrence of devastating effects called consequences. For example, it could lead to tissue breakdown and then severe hemorrhage (heavy release of blood) from a slipped ligature. As medical personnel, you should know how dangerous that is. Hence, there is a great need to take the writings on surgical knots very seriously, as we will be diving into knots in this chapter.

Before we dive into the various kinds of suture techniques, students of paramount importance should become skilled and fluent in tying various kinds of knots. There are two distinct approaches to tying these knots, either by hand or by making use of the instrument. When using your hands, the hand knots can be placed with either both hands or with a single hand.

Anatomy Of the Knot

This has to do with the composition of the surgical knot, as it is with human anatomy. There are fundamental components worthy of note regarding surgical knots, and these components are not to be taken for granted a bit. They tell you what and how of the knot. A surgeon is as good as his knot, so this part of the study cannot be neglected. Regardless of whatever method is used, one thing you should be aware of is that every knot of whatsoever kind consists of two kinds of loops. The first and most fundamental loop is the approximation loop. The probity of the suture is greatly dependent on this first loop. If this loop is not successfully placed, then you can declare your suture useless. The manner in which the loop must be placed should be in a way that, when pulled together, the two separate edges of the wound are maximized, in other words, approximated. The next loop, known as additional loops, is all referred to as termed securing loops. They aid in securing the whole knot, shielding from factors that will want to tamper with the knot.

Properties Of an Ideal Knot

In this section, you will be taken on a journey regarding the features an ideal knot should possess. The reason for these features is to prevent the knot from loosening, guard against an ineffective suture, and avoid compromising the overall result. We, by now, from preceding chapters, know how vital an ideal knot is to an effective suture. For the knot to be ideal, it must have both; Loop Security and Knot security.

1. **Loop security:** An insecure knot can lead to an obstructed view during the procedure if bleeding is not controlled, causing a postoperative hemorrhage, leading to hematoma. In addition, it is a fact that inadequate security can result in a knot that may project from the surface and can cause issues with wound healing, patient discomfort, and suboptimal

cosmetic appearance. In avoiding this, we are looking at loop security. This is a technique to overcome the loosening of surgical knots. It refers to the capacity or dexterity to ensure the future is firmly held together while the knot is being tied. Security of the knot depends on the materials used, the depth and location of the wound, and the amount of pull placed on the wound postoperatively.

2. Loop security can only be influenced by the knot tying technique. This implies that the security of a loop is solely dependent on the technique for knot tying in use. The surgical knots not properly tied may be loose, which may result in low loop security. For the security loop to be at its best, the suture material must be held taut between each throw.

3. **Knot Security:** This focuses on the integrity of the final knot. That is the concluding knot for the suture. Unlike loop security that is dependent on the knot tying technique, there are several factors that affect knot security.

These factors are as follows:

> Structural Configuration of the Knot: The square knot, which is thrown in opposite directions, has better knot security than the granny's knot, which is thrown in the same direction. Knots moving in opposite directions provide better knot security.

> The Type of Suture Material in use: Suture materials consisting of low "memory" and coefficient of friction tend to offer better knot security. The very ones with high coefficients may require extra throws to prevent loosening.

The memory has to do with the propensity of suture materials to recover their initial form and shape after deforming by tying. A material's high coefficient of friction affects the probity of the material, and therefore knot security can be compromised. The coefficient of friction is a measure of the slipperiness of the suture that affects the tendency of the knot to loosen after it has been tied.

> Suture End Length: There should be a suture end length of at least 3 mm after tying the knot to optimize knot security.

> ➤ Number of Throws: Certain materials require more throws to secure them. For materials such as nylon, polydioxanone, and polyglactin, there should be a minimum of three to five throws for optimum knot security. Progressive or running sutures must also be secured with more throws.

> ➤ Wound Environment: A fatty environment is bad for knot security, and this should be counterbalanced by a higher number of throws.

> ➤ Suture Diameter: Suture diameter is directly proportional to the knot security. This simply means that the security of a knot increases with an increase in suture diameter.

Principles Of Knot Tying

Basic microsurgical knot tying requires a series of manipulation of sutures with tying forceps (a handheld, hinged instrument used for grasping and holding objects.) under an operating microscope. The appropriate way of handling the forceps is of utmost importance in a successful knot tying. The tip of the forceps meant for tying should be used to lift the suture. Perhaps the suture material cannot be grasped; the tying platform should thoroughly be inspected for incomplete closure because of the damage to the platform or confinement of foreign matter. As over-compression in the case of music can lead to track distortion, so can the tight squeezing of the handle cause the tying platform to gape (open). Mastery of use in handling the suture material within the tying forceps is a fundamental step to successful knot tying in microsurgery.

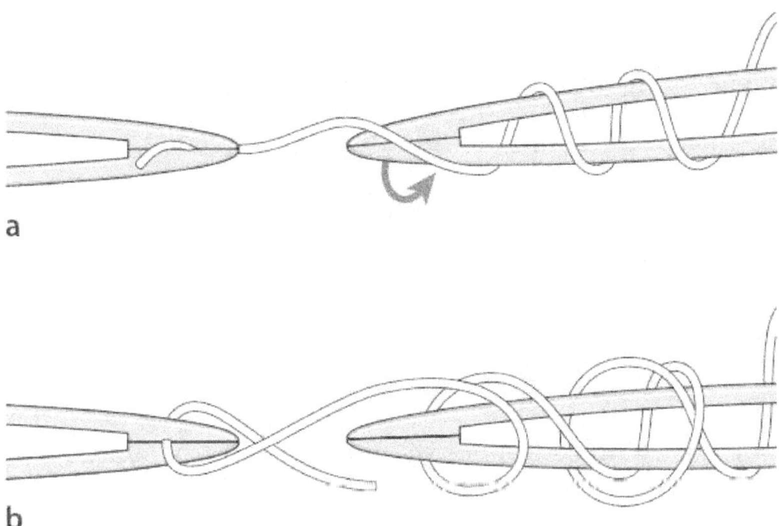

From the image above, there are some basic things to take note of:

a. Making the suture an extension of the forceps by loading longitudinally superiorly into the tying forceps. In this position, there is an increase in comfort with which the surgeon wraps the suture around the tying platform.

b. The suture is loaded diagonally in the tying platform. This method often makes wrapping the suture around another tying forceps more difficult and with little control.

When a suture is tied, it is expedient to position the edges (of the wound) beside each other. Basically, pressure should be exerted on the globe. Diverse knots may be used in executing this goal. One may be due to the rubbing together of the suture; in this case, the surgeon is careful to ascertain that the friction determines the knot tied. Poor slipknots result from rough threads. Smooth sutures, such as nylon, are easily knotted into slipknots. The basic principles of ophthalmic microsurgical knot tying include:

1. The choice of knot should be simple, pending on the circumstance.

2. The suture should be tied so that the wound edges are properly approximated (leaving no space).

3. Frequent back and forth movements should be avoided as much as possible as it results in friction that can weaken the material and cause it to break.

4. The first knotting loop, known as the approximation loop, performs the actual suturing function: It

connects and fixes the wound edges in the desired position (side by side). Every other additional loop serves only to secure the approximating loop.

5. Securing loops should be tightened at right angles to the suture plane so that they will not affect the established suture tension.

6. The approximation loop should not be tied too tightly, as it will contribute in no small way to tissue distortion or strangulation.

7. Extra throws do not add strength to a properly tied knot and only contribute to its bulk. A bulky knot can be difficult to bury. This means, in every way possible, one should avoid extra throws as they are of more harm than good.

8. The ability of a knot to hold depends largely on the friction created within the tightened loops (hence, the quality of the suture material plays an important role in knot construction):

   a. Rough suture materials are proper for square knots because of their high friction.

b. Smooth suture materials are adequate for slipknots because the approximating loop tends to loosen before the approximation loop is tied.

9. Regards for knot-tying technique is very important. Square knots and slipknots can be tied from the same initial loop arrangement. Only the direction of traction on the knots will determine which knot is created.

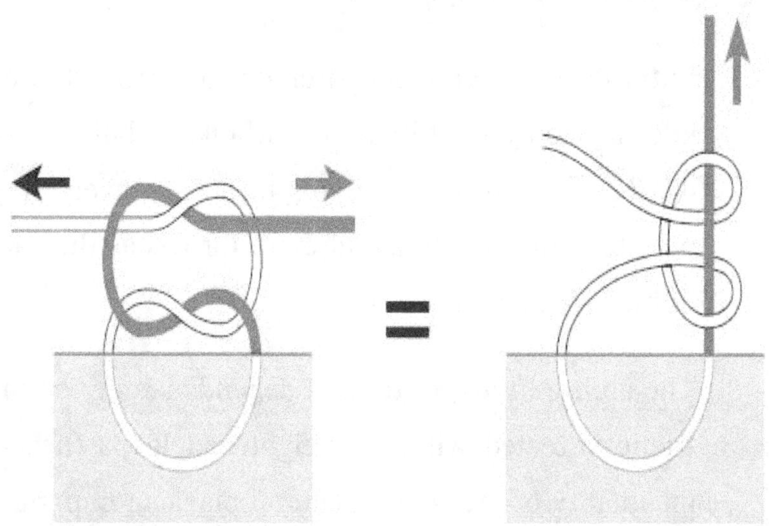

Caution must be taken to avoid the damage of the suture material when handling it. Avoid excessive manipulation of the suture with surgical instruments.

Excessive handling or twisting of the suture within the instrument may contribute to premature suture failure.

11. Surgical knots left on tissue surfaces are a source of irritation. Thus, knots must be as small as possible, and if the material is sufficiently tissue-compatible, they should be buried within the tissue.

12. The concluding knot must be as small as possible.

13. Ensure the concluding knot is properly in place with no chance of slipping off. If it is not, it should be redone rather than running at risk of wound breakdown.

Types Of Knots

Knots in the medical setting are used for securing bandages due to their binding effect. Depending on the type of suture you are using, each suture may have up to 3-4 knots in it. So there's a need for the knowledge of types of knots and how many knots are required to have a strong holding ability.

Let's look at the types of knots:

1. Square Knot:

This is simple to tie.

Method 1: Holding the rope of your stitches, you go left over right for one of the knots, then right over left for the other. The result should be an asymmetrical knot with two ends running parallel to each other.

Method 2: After stitches, leave one end of the stitches' thread longer than the other.

Step 1: Pass the long end over the needle holder in a clockwise direction, open the needle holder and grasp the small end, then pull it in.

Step 2: Make a loop in the anti-clockwise direction over the needle holder using the long end, then pull the short end in.

Step 3: Form another loop in the clockwise direction, repeat the process, and cut the end on the suture thread.

Disadvantage: Square knot is susceptible to slippage. The first bait is slipped, so there's a need for a second party to hold it firm or hold it yourself with your second hand.

Method 3:

Step 1: Assuming the two ends of the knots are in place. Place one end over the extended index finger and the rope resting on the left hand, while the second end of the rope is on the right hand.

Step 2: The second end/strand is fixed between the left thumb and index finger, still holding the first strand in the left hand.

Step 3: Left thumb swung in the first strand to make the first loop.

Step 4: Pass the second strand across the first strand and hold it between the left thumb and index finger.

Step 5: Push the second strand inside the first with the left hand and pull it out with the right hand. Pull in both directions to tighten the first hitch.

Step 6: Release the left index finger from the first strand and wrap the strand around the thumb. Hold the second strand with a right hand and push to the left slightly.

Step 7: Put the second strand between the left thumb and index finger. The second strand crosses over the first strand.

Step 8: First-strand slides into the left index finger to form a loop as the second strand is grasped between the left thumb and index finger.

Step 9: left thumb pushes the second strand into the first strand, then pulls out with the right hand. Pull in the opposite direction and form the second hitch.

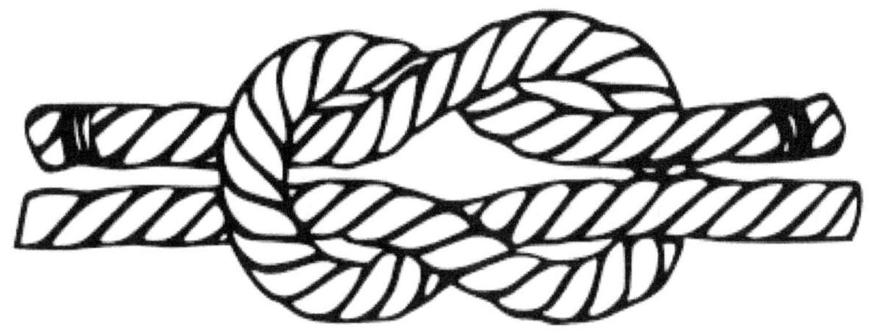

2. Surgeons Knot:

Step 1: Place the first strand over the extended index finger of the left hand and hold it in the left palm. Place the second strand within the thumb and index finger.

Step 2: Make the second strand cross the first strand still extended over the index finger of the left hand. Both fingers of the left hand come together.

Step 3: Loop of first-strand slips into the left thumb. The second strand grasps between the thumb and index finger.

Step 4: Second strand pushed inside first strand's loop by the index finger of the left hand. Pull in opposite directions.

Step 5: The loop formed is slid into the next thumb. The second strand is held between the left thumb and index finger.

Step 6: The index finger pushes the second strand inside the first loop and is pulled out by the right hand. Pull in the opposite direction.

Step 7: With the two ends (first strand and second strand). Put first-strand across the left thumb and in the left hand. Pass the second strand across the first and hold between the left thumb and index finger.

Step 8: Push the second strand in with the thumb. Pull in opposite directions.

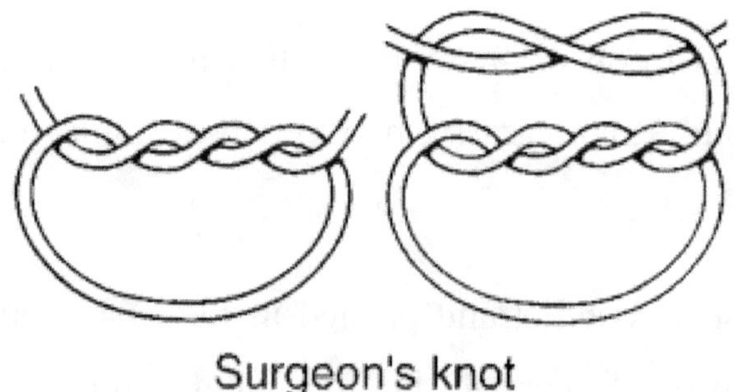

Surgeon's knot

3 Granny Knot:

Step 1: Hold the two ends of the strand in each hand. Cross the leftover right to make a loop. Then tie.

Step 2: Cross the left of right again and make another loop, then tie.

Step 3: It's prone to slippage, so the ends of the strand should be pulled in the opposite directions tightly and should be perpendicular to the load-carrying part of the strand.

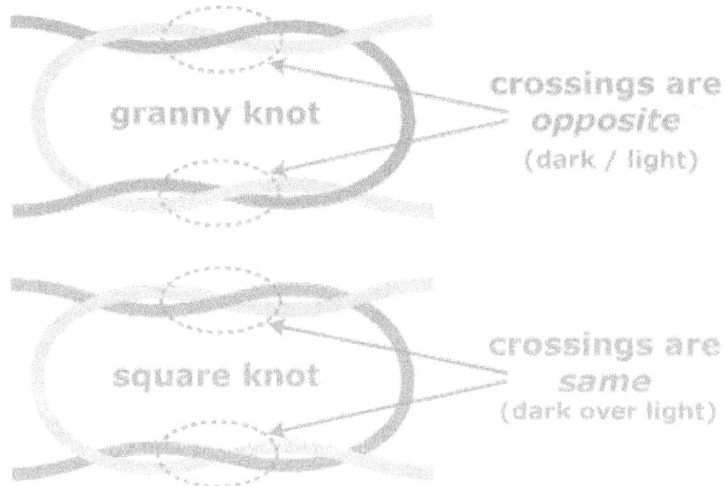

4. Slip Knot:

Step 1: Hold the two ends of the strand in a U-shape.

Step 2: Wind the long end over the top of the short end. Hold the point where the strand crosses tightly between your right thumb and index finger.

Step 3: Using your left hand, pick up the remaining body of the long end and form a loop similar to the first.

Step 4: Slip the second loop in the first. This will form a looped loop or loop in a loop.

Step 5: Pull the tail of the loop, i.e., the two ends of the strand (short and long end) to tighten the loop.

Step 6: Pull the two ends in opposite directions and tie, forming a slip knot.

5. Miller's Knot:

Step 1: Hold the strand over the stitches. Make an "X" of both long and short ends, the long end on top, and hold in between the left thumb and index finger.

Step 2: With the loop formed by crossing the strands. Slide the needle holder in with your right hand, grab the short end, cross over the long end, and then hold between the left thumb and index finger.

Step 3: Slide the needle holder within the loop, grab the short end, and pull it inside the loop using your right hand. Pull the ends in opposite directions.

Step 4: Make a loop around the needle holder, then pull the short end in and tie. This is to secure the ligature.

Step 5: Make a loop around the needle holder similar to the first and pull the short end in. Repeat the process four times. To make it tight and form a four-square knot.

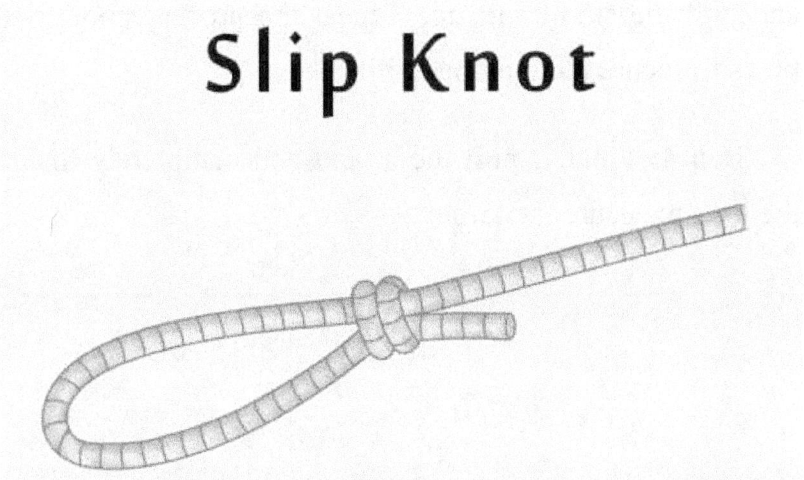

6. Aberdeen Knot:

This is an alternative to the square knot. It's also similar to a quick-release stitch used to tie a horse. It's a knot and the end of a suture line when the surgeon is left with a loop and the strand end.

Step 1: Hold the suture loop open and slide your right hand in it, holding the tail of the strand in the left hand.

Step 2: Pull the tail of the rope inside the loop with your right hand, then tighten it by pulling the loop and strand end in opposite directions (by maintaining traction on the working end).

Step 3: Slide your right hand through the loop again and pull the strand end in. Repeat the process about 4-8 times to secure the binding ability.

Step 4: Finally, pull the strand end completely inside the loop to secure the knot.

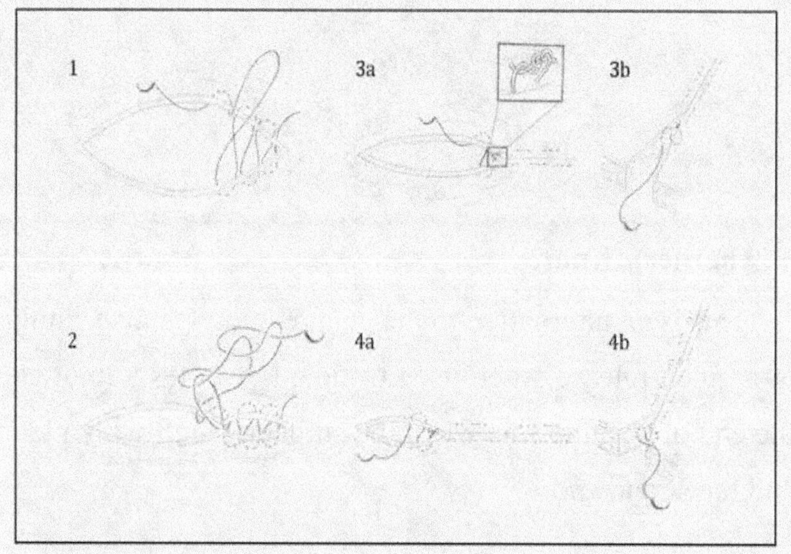

7. Half-Blood Knot:

This is one of the easiest but weakest knots. The half-blooded knot has been in usage for years back with no issues of extensor mechanism in elective replacements.

Tips

- Almost 100 percent strength is achieved when the knot is properly tied.
- Forceps and hemostats also perform the tying function.
- It is also known as a double surgeon's knot because of its activity of passing through the knot two times.
- The triple surgeon's knot makes use of three turns for added security. In the same view, it can be given 4,5 or 6 turns, increasing the complexity and bulkiness but adding strength.
- Almost the same technique is applied for tying the surgeon's end loop that can be joined to a swivel.

Method 1:

Four-stage techniques are required in tying a half-blooded knot with a tuck.

Stage 1: The suture is to be passed through the tissue to arrive at having two ends. The standing end should be properly held afterward. In this stage, a wide circle with the needle holders facing the wound is to be applied. Wind them four times about the thread in a similar way that a fender would be used with a sword.

Stage 2: Hold the working end, pull it through the loops of the thread being used. The thread should be pinched between the thumb and forefinger where the two free ends meet.

Stage 3: With the working end still being held, pass the needle holders through the triangular loop and then through the created loop.

Stage 4: Withdraw the needle holders while releasing the working end. Graph again with no pressure on the end as the standing end is pulled tight. Possibly, the needle holders can be used as a knot pusher.

Deliberation

The half-blooded knot with a tuck is mostly used in fishing to attach the line to hooks. NB: There is the possibility of slippage and weakness of the suture material in a surgical knot. However, as the half-blooded knot will not slip in contrast to a surgical knot, the tall can be cut shorter, thereby reducing the total material left in the wound.

Method 2:

Step 1: Holding the two ends of the strand after stitches in a U-shape, curve the long end and short end.

Step 2: Wrap the short end around the long end in a clockwise manner in six throws, forming a small loop close to the stitches.

Step 3: With your left hand, slide the small strand after forming the loop into the small loop.

Step 4: Pull the small strand out with the right hand and the long strand with the left. Pull gently to secure the knot.

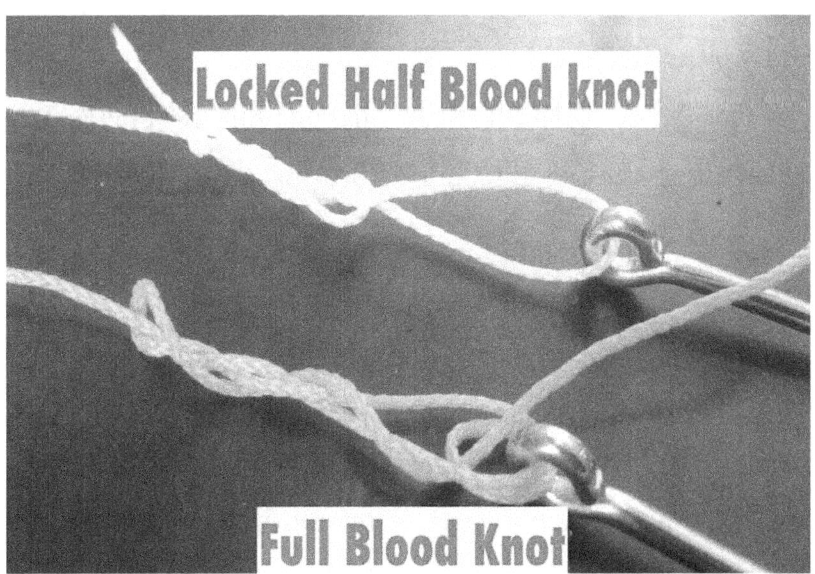

8. Forwarder Knot

Step 1: Holding the two ends of the strand. Cross one strand over the other to form number four.

Step 2: This forms a loop, then slips the crossed strand inside the loop and pulls out.

Step 3: Cross the strands again and tie just like the first. This is the forwarder Knot.

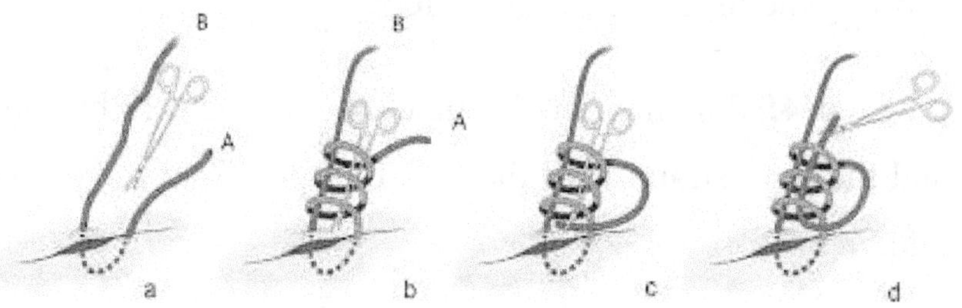

9. Delmar Knot:

This knot is particularly useful during endoscopic procedures, for example, during arthroscopy.

Step 1: With the needle holder in your dominant hand, make a loop with the long part of the suture material beside the suture needle.

Step 2: You will be able to pass the end of the suture material over the loop with your non-dominant hand. Do so.

Step 3: Make 2 to 3 more twists.

Step 4: Tighten the knots by pulling the free end with your needle holder.

10. Constrictor Knot:

This is a knot similar to the clove hitch but stronger than the clove hitch. It's a simple knot to ties

Step 1: Wrap your working end around your anchor twice, i.e., make your stitches around the anchor.

Step 2: Slide the working end into the loop where the two wraps meet. Then pull.

Step 3: Pull tightly to secure the knot. Unlike the clove-hitch, it won't work itself loose.

Complications Associated with Sloppy Suture

Usually, after intense hours of suturing, most medical personnel first ensure that the stitches will not cut loose rather than the wound care in general. However, even the professional personnel fear the stitches might loosen, especially when it's time to close the wound. The most important thing to note is that suturing a wound is a procedure that needs to be done carefully and avoid any errors. There are many ways a suture can come undone after surgery, and when this kind of event happens, there is a high tendency of infection to occur, which can lead to serious complications and sometimes death.

Most of the time, when sloppy suture occurs, it is often regarded as negligence on the medical personnel's part, and this act is considered medical malpractice.

Causes Of Sloppy Suture

When a suture is unfinished, this condition is termed wound dehiscence. This is the common complication of suturing, and it occurs when a wound opens along the suture.

Normally, a suture is supposed to remain in place until new tissues are formed and help the wound heal, so when wound dehiscence occurs, the sutured end opens instead of close to heal. There are many things that can cause sloppiness of suture.

Below are a few causes of sloppy suture:

<u>Excessive wound tension:</u> When a wound tension is excessive, it increases the risk of dehiscence and can lead to further complications.

<u>Foreign objects:</u> When there is the presence of a foreign object like needle, hair, or even cloth fibers in the site of suturing, it can cause sloppy sutures, and this can cause severe damage if not treated immediately.

<u>Infection in the wound:</u> Generally, infections affect the body. Colonization of viruses and bacteria leading to infections in a suturing site can also cause sloppy sutures, and if not treated immediately, can lead to severe damage.

<u>Incorrect knot:</u> When there is incorrect placement of a needle holder, it may result in a serious complication. Physicians need to understand and master each knot and know where to use it because knots help in maintaining appropriate tension in a wound which is important when it comes to proper healing.

<u>Tying knots too tight or loose:</u> A loose knot can lead to a serious complication. It can lead to the loosing of tension in a suture which can result in the suture opening and can also lead to snagging of the patient during their daily activities, and healing ability will be compromised. Also, when the knots are tight in excess, it can also lead to severe damage, it can lead to breakage of the incision, which can also lead to the potential cutting of tissues in the process.

<u>Placing of suture too close to wound edge:</u> When there is improper placement of sutures, the wound edge might experience inflammation, swelling, increased blood supply, and decreased collagen structure. Dead tissues can also be present, which can lead to suturing coming apart.

<u>Incorrect use of materials:</u> Mastering suturing instruments is important in the aspect of suturing. In a situation where there is an inappropriate use of material mismatching the suturing materials, the suture surely be undone and sloppy, and this can lead to severe damage.

<u>Early removal of sutures:</u> When the suture is removed before the appropriate time or is left for too long severe damage can occur. When the suture is removed before due time, the tissues beneath will not have time to bond, and the wound will open, which can lead to damage to the newly formed tissue, and this can give access to bacteria and viruses to the site of injury. And it is also important to remove the suture at the appropriate time without any extension because this can lead to excessive scarring.

<u>Blood Clot forming:</u> Blood is supposed to be circulating, but when it clots, especially in the site of injury, it can cause severe damage.

Symptoms of sloppy suture

A suture is meant to join the edges of the wound together, but sometimes it can become infected.

Below are some noticeable symptoms of a sloppy suture

- ✓ Redness in the suturing area.
- ✓ Swollen lymph nodes near the suture location.
- ✓ Feeling pain when someone touches the area or after movement.
- ✓ Feeling of warmth around the suturing site.
- ✓ Bad odor coming from the suturing site.

Risk Factors

Generally, nothing happens without a particular reason. When there is negligence from a patient, suturing can become sloppy, and sometimes it can be sloppy due to natural causes, e.g., overweight, compromised immune system, and a diabetic patient. A suture can become sloppy in people that smoke, this kind of people are also at high risk of not healing fast.

How To Prevent Sloppy Suture

While many factors can cause sloppiness of suture, there are a lot of ways to prevent its occurrence:

<u>Keeping the wound dry:</u> It is important to keep a wound dry, especially within the first 24hours after suturing. The presence of any kind of moisture can slow the healing process.

<u>Keeping the suture clean:</u> A suture is supposed to be kept clean always without the presence of any dirt. This can be done by avoiding all kinds of activities that may bring dirt or stain on the sutured area.

<u>Healing process:</u> A slight ooze might occur during the healing process, this is normal, and the scarring can be red, and this can fade with time.

<u>Pain relievers:</u> Taking paracetamol or Ibuprofen when there is mild pain can also help prevent the occurrence of a sloppy suture.

<u>Removal:</u> Removal of a suture at the appropriate time is also an important measure of preventing a sloppy suture. In some cases, the suture might fall before the due date, so seeking medical attention is important when this happens.

Scarring

A scar is a normal occurrence during the healing process. Every cut has to heal with a scar, but a scar can be less noticeable when proper care is taken during the healing process. Normally, a scar changes from thick to thin during the first 6-8 weeks after injury, and it can mature within the time of two years.

Looking After a Scar

Scar massage: A scar massage can be performed 2-4 weeks after injury. This can help in minimizing the visibility of the scar and also helps greatly in the healing process. But no massage should be done to an undone injury or an injury that is infected.

Moisturizing the scar: Moisturizers such as vitamin E and aloe vera can be used to soften a scar and for an easy-massage process.

Sun protection: It is also essential to prevent a scar from sun damage which can cause discoloration. A scar should always be covered with at least a sunblock or zinc cream. Clothing that covers the scar or the patient should always remain under a shade.

Daily activities: It is also essential to minimize some daily activities and avoid places with dirt like swimming pools and sandpits.

Problems Associated with A Scar

When a scar becomes painful or itchy, causes sleep disturbance, anxiety, and depression, there will be a need for mild or moderate treatment for it. For example, it can be treated using a Dermabrasion, a common medication for acne scar treatment, or injection that will make the scar smaller or flatter.

Complications Associated with Unabsorbable Suture

Suture Granuloma

This is a localized inflammatory reaction that occurs due to the retainment of suture materials.

This reaction usually develops after an intervention. It is characterized by a palpable and tender mass that resembles a tumor or recurrent tumor. They often occur in the unabsorbable suture and less in the absorbable; however, they sometimes occur.

QUICK EXERCISE 4

1. When a suture is unfinished, this condition is termed__________.

    A. Wound dehiscence B. Wound adherence C. Wound observance D. Wound requirement

2. ___________ is a localized inflammatory reaction that occurs due to retainment of suture materials.

    A. Suture Granuloma B. Suture glaucoma C. Suture granules D. Suture dehiscence

3. ___________is the common complication of suturing, and it occurs when a wound opens along the suture.

    A. Wound dehiscence B. Wound adherence C. Wound observance D. Wound requirement

4. _____________ changes from thick to thin during the first 6-8 weeks after injury, and it can take up to two years to mature.

A. Scar B. Suture glaucoma C. Suture granules D. Suture

5. _______________ can help in minimizing the appearance of the scar and also helps greatly in the healing process.

A. Scar massage B. Dryness C. Moisturizers D. Suture instruments

6. List the principles of an ideal knot.

7. List the types of suture knots.

CHAPTER 4
Techniques Of Suturing – Basic Sutures and Modification

As beginners, it is of utmost importance to know that, while suturing is a useful and commonly used surgical technique, knowing what method of sutures are needed and when they are not cannot be overemphasized.

Having had a grasp of what the previous chapters are all about, it is imperative for beginners to know the various techniques or methods and their modifications employed in carrying out sutures. In this chapter, these various basic techniques and their modifications will be thoroughly dealt with.

These basic techniques of suturing are:

1. Simple Interrupted Suture
2. Simple Running Suture

3. Vertical Mattress Suture

4. Horizontal Mattress Suture

5. Figure-of-8 Suture

6. Interrupted Cruciate Suture/Cruciate Mattress Suture

Simple Interrupted Suture

Simple Interrupted Suture is the basic standard suture (most fundamental technique) used for closure and epidermal approximation. It is the most commonly used technique in the closure of skin. It is known as an interrupted stitch because the individual stitches aren't connected; they are separate. In an interrupted suture, each stitch has its own knot. Its beauty is that the tension of each suture along the incision can be adjusted during the suturing.

Figure 1- Simple Interrupted Suture

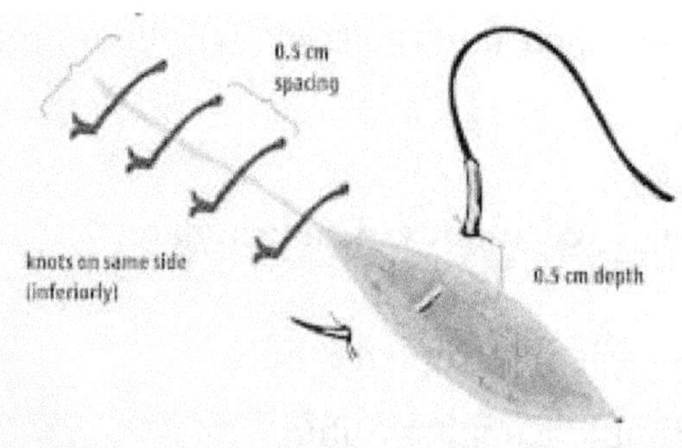

The needle is inserted in an initial site of the wound (about 5 mm of wound edge), then passed through the dermis depth, then the subcutaneous tissue to the opposite side for wound with close range to the wound edge, the knot is then tied close to the wound edge. This makes the final look of the suture cross-section flask-shaped. Making use of the thinnest suture possible is the best. This ensures that there are minimal suture tracts and also body reactions.

Note: Suture choice will depend largely on anatomic location and the goal of suture placement.

Equipment

1. Needle holder (driver) - To be held with the dominant hand.

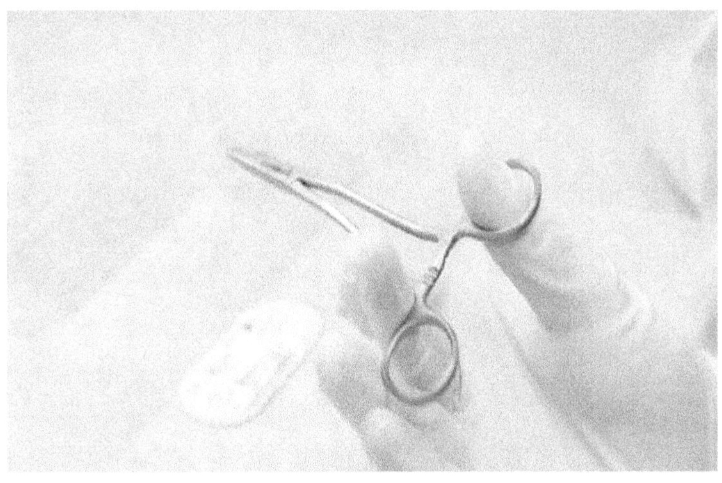

2. **Toothed forceps (pickups)**-To be held with the non-dominant hand.

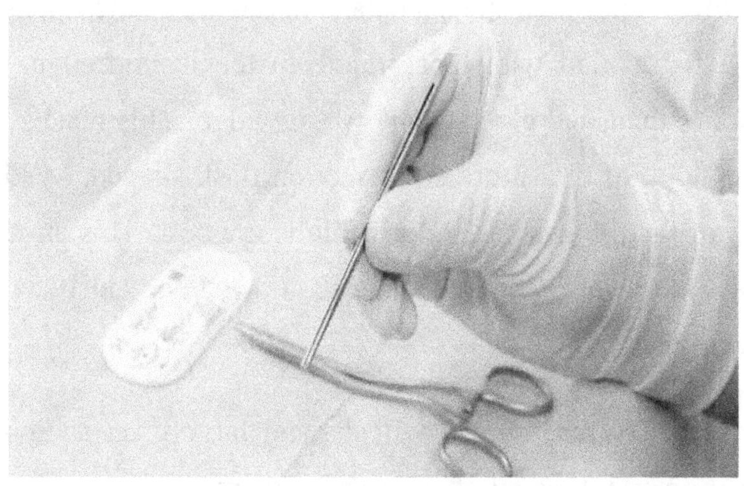

3. Scissors

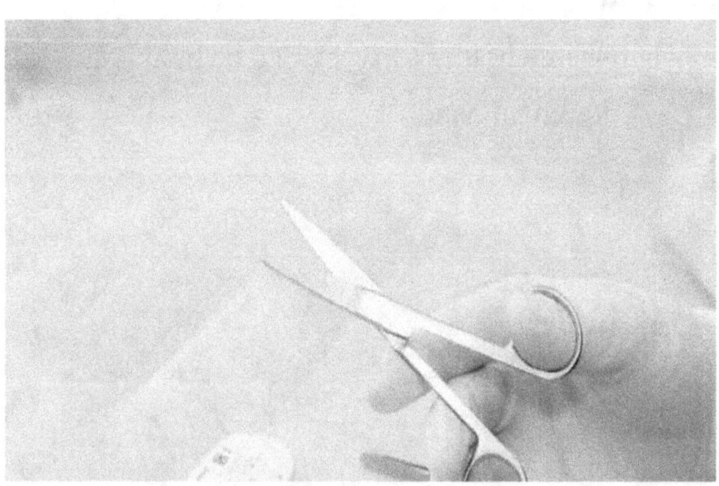

4. Suture

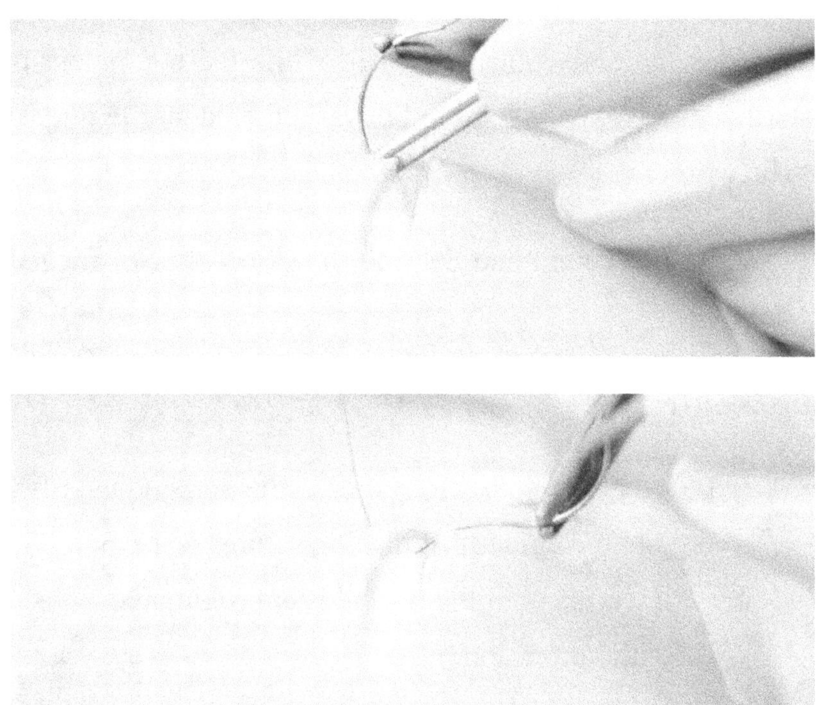

As beginners, it is appropriate to start a suture pattern using an approach that permits the comfortable use of surgical needles and instruments. Frequently, surgeons, depending on the orientation of a wound, can choose to place the needle from right to left or from left to right, top to bottom or bottom to top. All these are also functions of efficiency in knowing which pattern is appropriate in a case.

It is imperative to know that suturing as a process is a sterile procedure, and therefore the wound and surrounding skin must be antiseptically treated while the equipment is sterilized. Also, hands are to be washed, and sterile gloves to be worn.

Wash the wound and debride the skin edges of ragged or dirt.

Procedure:

1. To begin with, insert the needle perpendicularly into the epidermis, placing sutures at 1 cm intervals until the wound is approximated without tension.
2. With a fluid motion of the wrist, pass the needle through the dermis until it comes out of the middle of the wound.
3. With the aid of the forceps, gently hold and pull the needle upward while the needle holder is released.
4. With the aid of the forceps, raise the other edge of the wound and pass the needle perpendicularly through the dermis from inside to outside. Use the curvature of the needle and

fluid motion wrist to move the needle through the skin.

5. Now, as the needle surfaces on the outside, use the forceps to hold the needle and pull it through the skin.

6. Having Pulled the suture through the skin for about an approximate length of 3 cm on the opposing side, make a loop to the knot.

7. Repeat this process for consecutive sutures.

A. Simple Running Suture

Unlike the simple interrupted suture, in a simple running suture, the suturing process is continuous; that's is why it is also known as **Continuous suture.** Continuous stitches always start with what is called "Initial knot," which runs continuously to the end of the wound before the finishing knot is made. It is a technique useful for long wounds as it helps to minimize tension. It is also employed in securing a split or full-thickness skin graft. Using continuous sutures, fewer scars occur compared to interrupted sutures because fewer knots are made with simple running sutures, though the number of needle insertions is the same. In addition, speed is also one of the major advantages of the continuous suture technique in the sense that it does not require a knot at the end of each cross as required in Simple Interrupted Suture. All the stitches required to close a wound in running suture can be finished with one knot.

Equipment:

The same as listed above.

Procedure:

1. The first step: Gently lift the skin with forceps and pierce the skin surface with the needle perpendicular (90°) to the skin at approximately 4 mm from the wound edge.

2. An interrupted suture is made on one end of the edges of the wound, where the knot is tied in the same insertion direction. Leave a length of long suture that would be long enough to double back when making subsequent crosses.

3. At the other opening, the needle is reinserted along the wound as it penetrates the epidermis and passes through dermal or subcutaneous.

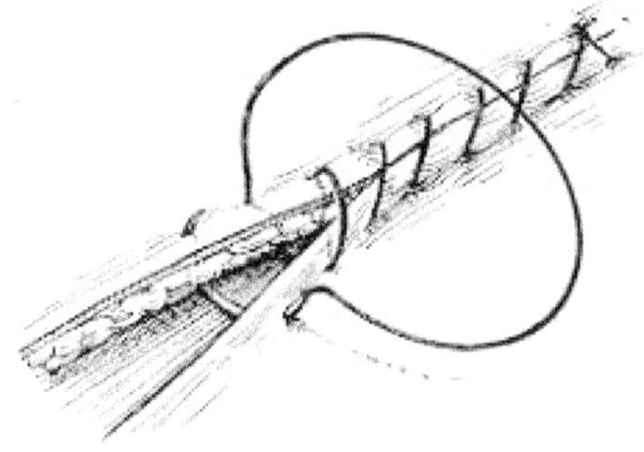

4. With the aid of the forceps, gently hold and pull the needle upward while the needle holder is released.

5. The needle is then driven through the full thickness of the skin by the fluid motion of the wrist to rotate the needle and pass it through the skin.

6. A loop is made, and the suture is tied off using square knots, just as if it were a simple interrupted stitch except, there is a trail of approximately 3-4 mm of strand after cutting off the shorter strand.

7. This process is repeated.

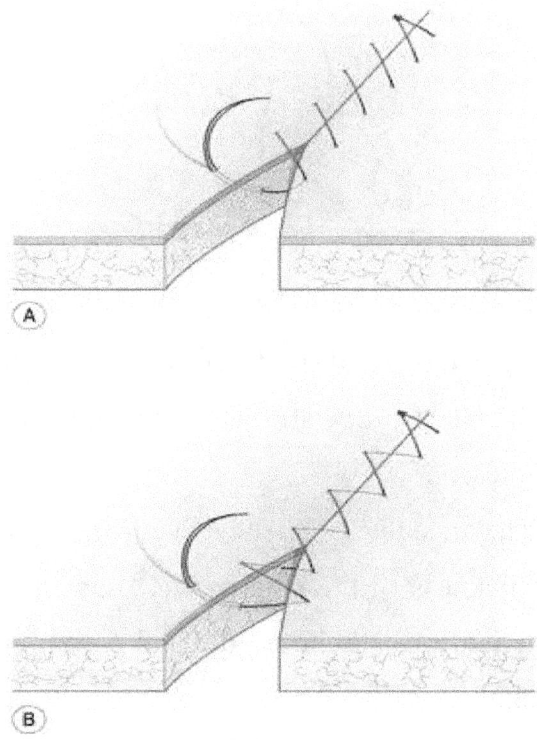

B. Vertical Mattress Suture

Vertical mattress Suture is a technique that is particularly effective for closing both deep and superficial tissue layers. In this method, instead of running the suture through each side of the wound and tying the ends off in a knot, the vertical mattress technique reinserts the needle closer to the wound, usually about 1 to 2 mm from the wound edge, bypassing across the wound twice at two different depths. A vertical mattress suture essentially serves as two sutures to achieve deep and superficial wound closure simultaneously. In a vertical mattress, the suture has one deep throw and one superficial throw (directly above and parallel) to evert the skin edges.

Equipment:

The same as listed above.

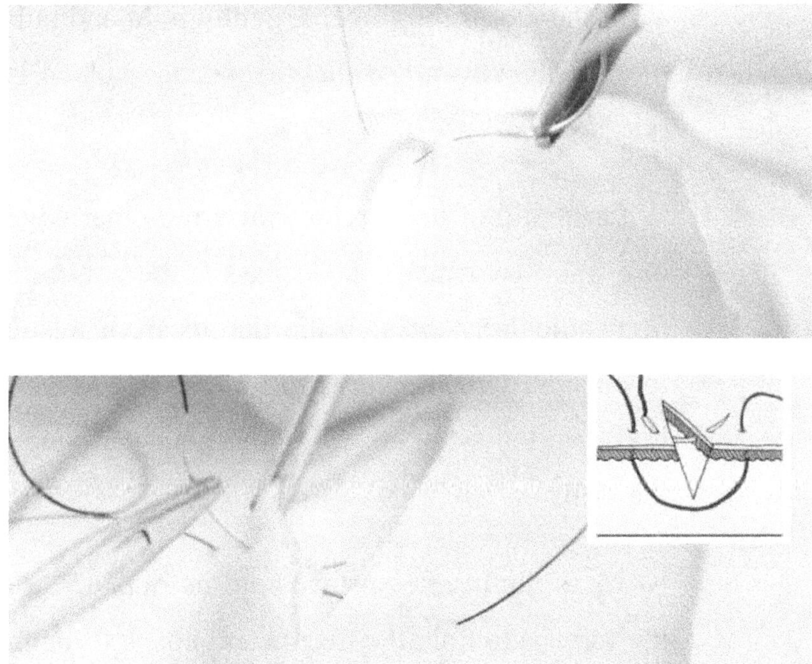

Procedure:

1. To begin with, gently lift the skin with forceps and pierce the skin surface with the needle perpendicular (90°) to the skin at approximately

4 mm from the wound until the wound is without tension.

2. With a fluid motion of the wrist, pass the needle through the dermis and until it comes out of the middle of the wound.

3. With the aid of the forceps, gently hold and pull the needle upward while the needle holder is released.

4. With the aid of the forceps, raise the other edge of the wound and pass the needle perpendicularly through the dermis from inside to outside. Use the curvature of the needle and fluid motion wrist to move the needle through the skin.

5. Now, as the needle surfaces on the outside, use the forceps to hold the needle and pull it through the skin.

6. Having Pulled the suture through the skin for about an approximate length of 3 cm on the opposing side, use the forceps to grasp the needle and pull it through the skin.

7. Ensure to follow the curvature of the needle as it travels through the skin and pulls the suture through as it goes. There should now be a suture crossing perpendicularly to the wound, approximately 3-4 mm from the wound edge.

8. Make another insertion, throwing another suture across the wound directly above or superficial to your original throw, taking smaller bites of the skin edge to evert the wound edges.

9. Continue to follow the curvature of the needle as it travels through the skin.

10. Make a loop and tie the suture off using square knots. Hold the suture end with the needle holder. Pull the needle holder in your direction and push the non-dominant hand away to lay the final knot. To avoid crushing the skin, do not pull the suture too tight.

11. The sutures should then be cut at about 5-6 mm long.

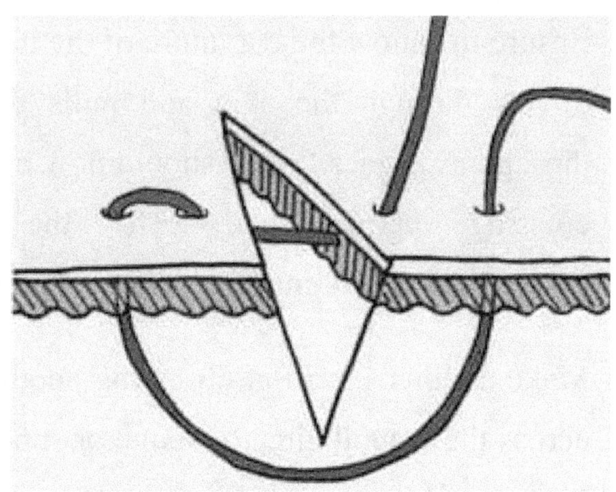

C. HORIZONTAL MATTRESS SUTURE

This suture is most found useful for temporary placement amidst a difficult repair with high tension. It also helps to evert wound edges in conditions where the skin is liable to naturally inverting into the wound. At times, it can be difficult to bring wound edges together to facilitate simple interrupted sutures. The placement of a horizontal mattress suture is employed to overcome this difficulty.

Equipment:

The same as listed above.

Procedure:

1. To start with, insert the needle perpendicularly into the wound, at about half the radius of the distance from the wound edge. Note that a larger

wound requires a larger-sized needle that would generally be about 1 cm from the wound edge.

2. With a steady move of the wrist joint, the suture needle is then loaded in a backhanded manner, and a second throw made approximately 1 cm down the wound edge on the same side, having a perpendicular entry into the wound and exiting on the side where you began.

3. Ensure to follow the curvature of the needle as it travels through the skin and pulls the suture through as it goes. There should now be a suture crossing perpendicularly to the wound, approximately 3-4 mm from the wound edge.

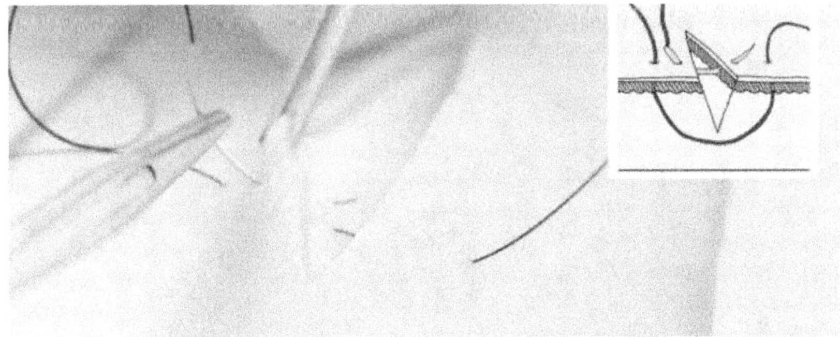

4. Make another insertion, with another suture across the wound superficial to your first throw,

taking smaller bites of the skin edge to turn out the wound edges.

5. A square box shape should be made at the end of this point.

6. At this point, loop the suture away around the needle holder twice, then grasp the suture end with the needle holder. Pull the needle holder in your direction and push the non-dominant hand away to lay the first knot.

7. Having dome that, loop the suture back towards you around the needle holder once and ensure the suture end is held with the needle holder. Abduct the needle holder and adduct your non-dominant hand to lay the second knot.

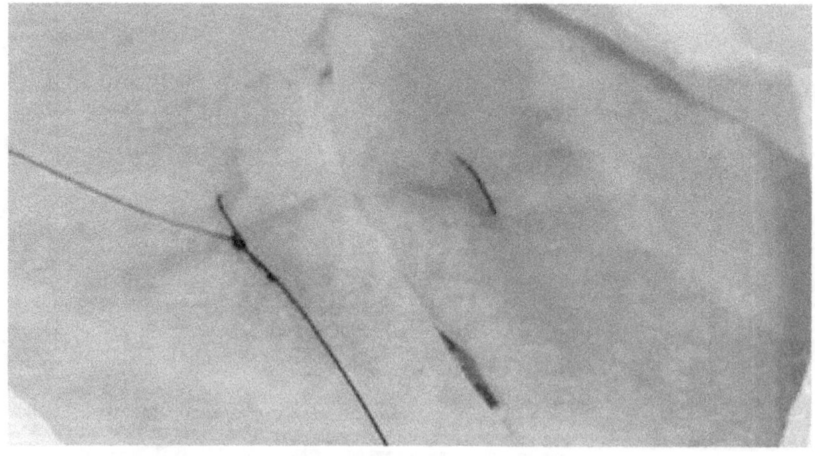

D. Figure-Of-8 Suture

"Figure of 8" suture is useful in areas where there is tension across the wound, and a single stitch might pull through the tissue.

It is usually composed of two access of the needle through the tissues, both directed towards the surgeon. The needle enters the epidermis (the skin), emerges beneath, and removes pronation, bringing directly across the side — in a mirror image fashion — to exit on the opposite side. Basically, the "Figure of 8" suture is a variation of the horizontal mattress suture with a lot of similarities. It also has some similarities with the simple interrupted technique. "Figure of 8" suture is often the most preferred among these two techniques. Its strongest or most common application is using it as a strong hemostasis suture where a good strength of stitch across the laceration would be achieved. This is seen in closing the uterus after a cesarean section and in neurosurgery when doing spinal column surgeries.

Equipment:

The same as listed above.

Procedure:

1. To start, gently lift the skin with forceps and insert the needle 90° to the skin at about 4 mm from the wound edge.

2. Plunge down and then rotate the needle with a fluid motion of your wrist joint so that the needle goes through the dermis and is brought out of the middle of the wound.

3. Use the forceps to hold the needle while the needle holder is being released.

4. Re-hold the needle just there with your needle holder.

5. Re-clamp so that you can go straight across the laceration with the same depth in the tissue and exit again from the surface of the epidermis with the same distance from the skin edges.

6. Now reload the needle the way you had loaded and go back across the same direction, just down the laceration a little bit.

7. Repeat what you just did. Note: It's a combination of both simple interrupted and horizontal mattress sutures.

8. A knot is then tied perpendicularly across the first cross, which gives this technique a 'Figure of 8'.

E. Interrupted Cruciate Suture/Cruciate Mattress Suture

Interrupted Cruciate Suture, also known as the **Cross-Mattress pattern**, is well efficient and stronger than the simple interrupted pattern because it resists tissue eversion.

It should be noted that cruciate suture is an infrequently used technique that is a hybrid between a simple interrupted suture, a mattress suture, and a simple running/continuous suture. It is useful when the benefits of interrupting sutures — most especially when the frequency of knot placement leads to a more secure closure —are needed. It may also be required when the wound length of a wound is too long for a single simple interrupted suture. This technique entails taking two simple interrupted bites in succession and then tying off the suture, leaving a cross pattern of suture material over the wound edge. It may also be used as an option in a secondary layer to facilitate the approximation of the epidermis when the dermis has been closed using any other method

Equipment:

The same as listed above.

Procedure:

1. To start, gently lift the skin with forceps and insert the needle through the skin surface at 90°, about 4 mm from the wound edge.

2. Plunge down and then rotate the needle with a fluid motion of your wrist joint so that the needle goes through the dermis and is lifted out of the middle of the wound.

3. Use the forceps to hold the needle while the needle holder is being released.

4. Re-hold the needle just there with your needle holder.

5. Re-clamp so that you can go straight across the laceration with the same depth in the tissue and exit again from the surface of the epidermis with the same distance from the skin edges.

6. The cruciate suture is finished by tying an instrument knot with a double first throw followed by single throws. The knot is placed by the inside of the incision.

Shaky Hands or Hand Tremor

Surgery can be stressful, and no matter how skillful one is, sometimes there is the presence of anxiety which can bring tremors. But this anxiety can be managed because tremors in a theatre room can lead to severe complications, sometimes death. The level of tremor manifesting when a person is in a resting position is different from one that occurs when someone is performing a complex tax like suturing. The effect of tremors can affect the quality and duration of surgery in most cases. But most people assume that medical personnel are the coolest and calmest people in the world, making everything look easy. But the important thing to note is, no one is perfect, and nobody is above mistakes. Surgeons do feel anxiety, and mostly they make it under control to the extent that it becomes unnoticeable.

Do surgeons have steady hands?

Most medical professionals have steady hands, which comes from routine practice, experience, and confidence.

But trainees' surgeons that are just starting are bound to experience such due to lack of experience and anxiety. This mainly occurs due to nerves and lack of practice. But these things reduce with time and exposure. And also, some medical schools take this aspect important, and they offer programs that assess potential surgeons in this aspect.

Types Of Hand Tremor

Hand tremor is classified into two:

- Physiological tremor
- Pathological Tremor

Causes Of Hand Tremor

Anxiety: This is the common and physiological cause of hand tremors. Under physiological conditions, anxiety can be controlled, and mostly, with practical routine, it becomes unnoticeable and does not affect the surgical procedure.

Essential Tremor: This is one of the common reasons why medical personnel experience shaky hands in the surgical room. Most of the time, when the symptoms are minimal, it is unnoticeable and won't affect everyday tasks or job. But when the symptoms become severe, it may affect the job, and one will need medicine, therapy, or surgery. In this case, when medical personnel suffer from essential tremor, which is severe, it can affect the quality of surgery; such a person cannot even be allowed to perform any operation.

Medical Personnel with Parkinson's Disease

Parkinson's disease occurs when brain cells that control muscles movement get damaged. When a medical person is diagnosed with this condition, it may affect the quality of their profession because this kind of person will have trouble in balance, stiffness of the hands and legs. This kind of person cannot also be allowed to perform any medical operation to avoid any complications.

Multiple Sclerosis: This is a condition characterized by damage in a coating on a nerve called myelin. When this occurs, the symptoms include shaky hands, and when medical personnel is diagnosed with this condition, they are mostly asked to minimize medical procedures due to the risk associated with it.

Hyperthyroidism: Shaky hands might often be a sign of an increasing level of secretion of thyroid hormones. When medical personnel experience these symptoms and are diagnosed with the disorder, they are mostly asked to put a halt in entering the operation room.

Caffeine: Taking a cup or two of coffee isn't a new thing. Coffee contains caffeine, a stimulant, and in as much as it is a stimulant, it can make hands shaky when you have too much of it (caffeine overdose). Caffeine can also be found in almost all soda drink which we consume daily and have become the order of the day now. When medical personnel show symptoms of this disease, performing surgery by them can cause severe complications and damage.

Huntington's disease: This is a condition characterized by the breaking down of the brain's nerve cells. It affects emotions, cognitive abilities, and physical movement. It causes hallucination, involuntary movement, depression, and difficulty making decisions. A medical person with Huntington's cannot be allowed to carry out a procedure on a patient as they also need medical attention.

Vitamin deficiency: Vitamins like vitamin B12, B-6, or B-1 are essential for maintaining the nervous system. The deficiency of such vitamins can lead to shaky hands.

Risk Factors Associated with Hand Tremor

Any mistake or intentional action during surgery can lead to severe complications and damage and sometimes can cost the patient's life.

How To Manage or Get Rid of Hand Tremor

1. When there is an underlying condition causing the tremor like hyperthyroidism, then the underlying condition needs to be treated. When the underlying cause is treated, then the tremor stops.

2. There are cases where the tremor is a side effect. In cases like this, there is a need to switch medications.

3. Avoiding substances that cause tremors like caffeine can reduce or stop the tremor.

4. Using physical therapy to enhance the control of muscles. There are a lot of occupational therapists that engage people with tremors.

5. When anxiety is the cause of tremors, there is a need for relaxation and meditation practices that help relieve such anxiety or panic.

6. In cases of essential tremor, anti-seizure medication, or beta-blockers.

7. When parkinsonism is the cause, drugs like levodopa and carbidopa are used to manage the condition.

8. There are some tremors with no obvious cause. In such cases, tranquilizers are used.

QUICK EXERCISE 5

1. List five methods on how to manage tremor hands.

2. Most medical professionals have steady hands, which comes as a result of?

    A. Routine practice B. Multiple sclerosis C. Parkinson's disease D. Not practicing

3. _______________ is a technique that is particularly effective when it comes to closing both deep and superficial tissue layers.

    A. Vertical mattress suture B. Horizontal mattress suture C. Simple mattress suture D. Parallel mattress suture

4. __________ is a type of suture that is mostly found useful for temporary placement amidst a difficult repair with high tension.

A. Vertical mattress suture B. Horizontal mattress suture C. Simple mattress suture D. Parallel mattress suture

5. ____________ suture is finished by tying an instrument knot where there is a double first throw, followed by single throws.

A. cruciate B. Hybrid C. Simple C. Horizontal

6. List five causes of hand tremors.

CHAPTER 5
Techniques Of Suturing – Advanced Suture

Hybrid Suture:

This suture is effective in terms of faster healing of collagen infiltration between the yarns and individual filaments. It serves as a mix between the vertical mattress and horizontal mattress techniques. It's usually used solely for wounds under minimal tension. Techniques involving this suture includes:

1. The suture needle is inserted approximately 4 mm from the wound edge perpendicular to the epidermis.

2. The needle takes a wider bite of the dermis because of the curvature nature at 4 mm from the wound edge and emerges on the contralateral side at the same level as the first insertion on the epidermis.

3. The needle is then reinserted in a backhand fashion perpendicular to the epidermis on the same side and the same level of the incision line as the just exited epidermis contralateral to the epidermis relative to the surgeon.

4. The needle then takes a bite of the dermis at the same 4 mm distance to the wound edge.

5. The needle then exits through the epidermis relative to the surgeon.

6. The process is then continued throughout the wound length.

7. A knot is then applied to the suture material carefully to minimize tension across the epidermis and avoid causing a tear to the tissue.

Dermal/ Subcuticular Sutures

This is an intradermal suturing procedure where sutures don't rupture the skin but remain in the dermis, and as such, no marks are seen on the skin. Subcuticular suturing requires a non-contaminated, even edges wound in the dermal layer of the skin, and for this reason, it's most common in operating rooms but rarely employed in the emergency room. Steps required to carry out this suturing includes:

1. Starting either to the left or right of the apex, place the needle in a parallel plane to the incision. Take a bite through the skin surface a few mm above the wound and out through the dermis parallel to the incision line. Tie down the suture with an instrument tie or adhesive bandage.

2. Cross the needle over to the side from which the first bite was taken and insert it a little further at the same level of the first bite and pull it through the dermis on the other side to emerge a little further along the wound length, maintaining the same parallel orientation.

3. Continue the process until the end of the wound is reached.

4. Once the last horizontal bite is taken, leave some slack in the suture, pull the distal material through, and hold it firmly, making it your loop.

5. Use this new loop to tie down a continuous stitching knot.

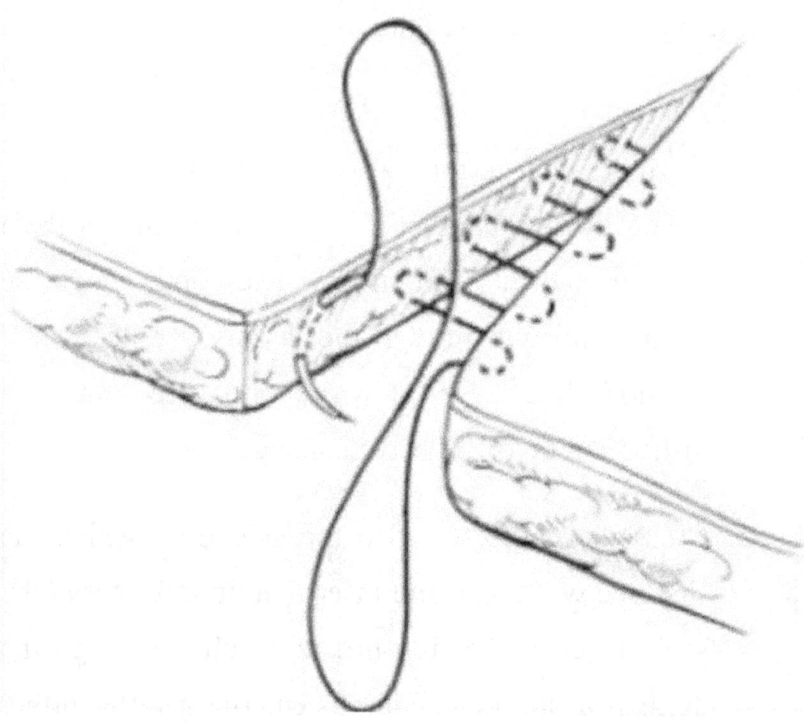

Purse-String Suture

This type of suture is so-called because it resembles the string drawn to close the mouth of a coin purse.

Purse-String suture is defined as a surgical suture passed as a running stitch in and out along a circular wound edge in such a pattern that when the ends of the suture are drawn tight, the wound closes like a purse. The suture is used to provide primary closure for small skin defects or as a partial closure for larger round lacerations.

It's frequently used by surgeons as closure for cuticle defects.

To carry out this procedure, the following steps will be taken:

1. Round skin markings for surgical removal of the lesion are done around the wound.

2. An absorbable suture is used. The suture enters and exists intradermally (i.e., the needle enters the superficial surface and goes out through the deep surface) and never penetrates the epidermis in a circular pattern.

3. The needle should always be inserted at an equal distance from the dermal exit site.

4. This procedural sequence should be continued until all the marked surgical area is sutured.

5. When the initial entry and final exit points meet, the suture is pulled with increasing strength and then tied gently to close the skin defects completely. Once the closure is completed, a suture knot is tied within the wound. No external stitches are necessary.

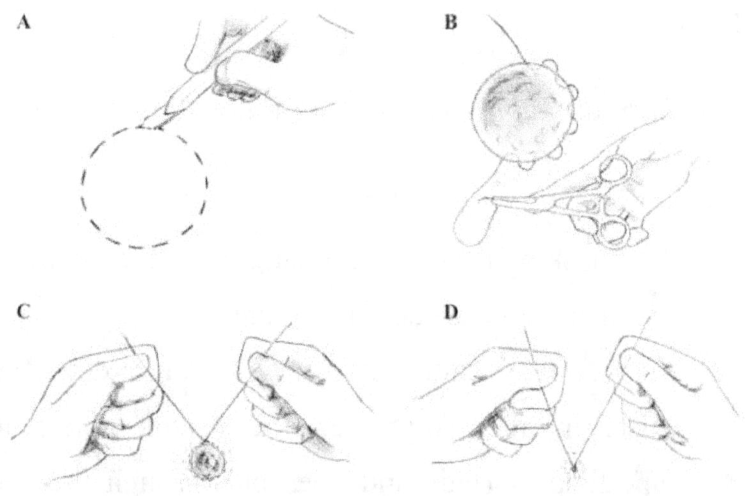

Winch Suture

This suture is used for wounds under a significant amount of tension. When closing wounds under marked tension, transepidermal pulley sutures may be inadequate to close the wound totally. As a result, a temporary winch suture is employed in order to hold tissues in approximation while other sutures are put in place.

This suture is intraoperatively removed after other tension-relieving sutures have been employed.

Techniques involved in winch suture include:

1. The needle is inserted at 90^0 to the epidermis of the first wound edge at a distance away from the wound.

2. It passes through the dermis and pierces the dermis of the second wound edge, and comes out on the contralateral side on the same level as the first wound edge.

3. The loose ends of the suture material are then secured with a hemostat (an instrument that clamps broken blood vessels to diminish the blood flow).

4. The first wound edge is then pierced again at the same level as the preceding suture, passes through the dermis and pierces the dermis of the opposing edge, or second wound edge, and comes out on the contralateral side.

5. This procedure is repeated throughout the entire wound length.

6. The long suture material is then cut off at the end of the procedure, leaving a few centimeters. The hemostat is removed from the first loose end and tied together with a few centimeters from the just-cut edge.

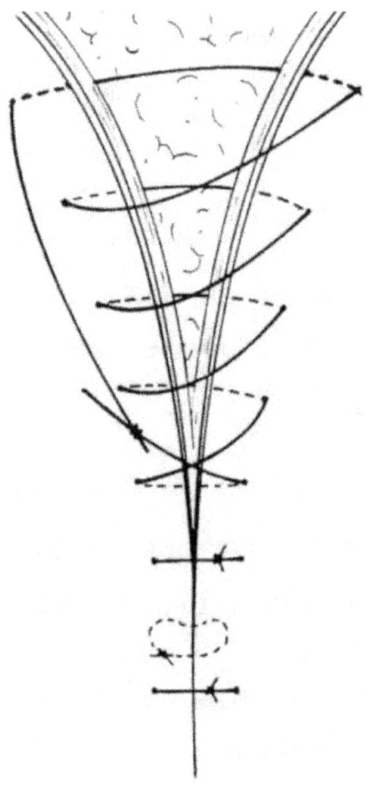

Cross Suture

This is a simple running stitch procedure used for closure, hemostasis (i.e., keeping blood in a damaged blood vessel to stop bleeding), and a close approximation of wounds.

Techniques involved include:

1. The needle is inserted at 90^0 to the epidermis at a distance from the wound edge and pulled out on the contralateral side at an even distance from the wound edge with the first insertion.

2. Surgical forceps on the left hand is used to grasp the needle body on the contralateral side and pull it upwards as the body of the needle on the other end is released from the needle drive.

3. At this point, there's a loose end of the suture material left. It can be held with a hemostat to prevent pulling when suturing.

4. To continue suturing, the suture material left at the initial insertion point is then used.

5. The needle is inserted on the contralateral side like a simple running stitch and pulled. It's then taken back through the just left-wound edge dermis and pulled.

6. This process continues through the entire wound length.

7. Once the contralateral apex is reached, the leading end is now used to repeat (1) and (5), though, this time, the steps continue in the contralateral direction of the contralateral end along the wound, but the entry and exit points cross over the previously placed line of sutures forming an X appearance.

8. Once the beginning is reached, the hemostat is released, and the short end material is used to tie a reef knot. The remnant is now cut off.

Lembert Suture

This is the easiest technique that can be used for the internal organs, performed relatively quickly. It inverts the lips of the wound and never passes through the mucosa, therefore lowering the contamination probability. It is useful primarily to recreate a natural crease.

Techniques involved include:

1. The needle is inserted perpendicular at approximately 8 mm away from the wound edge.

2. The needle is rotated superficially through the dermis, and the needle tip exits 2 mm away from the wound edge on the ipsilateral side.

3. The needle is then taken over to the contralateral side and inserted 2 mm away from the wound edge.

4. The needle is then rotated superficially again through the dermis. It exits 8 mm away from the incised wound edge on the same contralateral side.

5.   A knot is then tied gently on the suture material, with care being taken to reduce tension across the epidermis.

Lattice Suture

This suture is used for the repair of excisional defects in the skin under tension or severely atrophic skin. This basic lattice stitch distributes tension away from the perpendicular plane of wound closure significantly more than a simple interrupted stitch.

Techniques involved include:

1.   Simple interrupted stitches, as taught in the previous chapter, are placed parallel to the wound edge on both sides. These simple interrupted stitches form the anchoring framework.

2.   To place the simple interrupted stitches, the needle is inserted at a distance to the wound edge of approximately 8 mm.

3.   The needle runs parallel to the incision line through the motion of the wrist, inserting it into the dermis and exiting it on the ipsilateral side. This process of insertion and exit parallel to the incision line runs through the entire wound length. The suture

material left after the simple interrupted stitch has been completed parallel to the incision line is then tied up loosely.

4. The needle is taken to the contralateral side, and steps (2) and (3) are repeated.

5. Incorporating the suture material from the anchoring framework, a simple interrupted suture is placed. The needle is placed perpendicular to the epidermis, lateral to the anchoring suture at a distance of approximately 2 mm to the anchoring suture.

6. The needle is inserted, runs through the dermis, and exits on the contralateral side at the same point lateral and at 2 mm distant to the anchoring suture.

7. A knot is tied off gently using the suture material. Care is taken when tying the knot to avoid straining the epidermis and constricting the suture.

Combined Vertical Mattress Dermal Suture

This combination suture may be seen as a hybrid between a vertical mattress suture and a dermal suture. It's a time-saving suture designed to permit the closure of multiple deep defects and simultaneously allow the eversion of wounds with the same suture.

Techniques involved include:

1. The needle is inserted at a 6 mm distance perpendicular to the wound edge.

2. The needle is rotated through the dermis, taking a deep bite and emerging at the center of the wound edge.

3. The needle is then inserted through the dermis of the incised wound edge and brought out on the contralateral side.

4. The needle is then crossed in a backhand fashion over to the ipsilateral side and inserted again. The needle takes a deep bite through the dermis and exits on the contralateral side at about 6 mm distance to the wound edge.

5. In a backhand fashion, the needle is inserted perpendicular to the epidermis at about 3 mm distant to the wound edge on the same contralateral side it exited from.

6. The needle emerges on the original side from which it was first inserted at a 3 mm distance to the wound edge.

7. The suture material is then tied off gently to avoid straining the wound edge and to avoid overly constricting the wound edges.

Kessler's Locking Loop

This process is used for tendons and ligaments.

Techniques:

1. The needle is inserted through the tendon from the deep to the superficial. It's then taken round the tendon from below, away from the operator.

2. The needle is inserted from the superficial side to the deep, thus forming a lock.

3. The needle is then taken over to the separated tendon and inserted from the deep to the superficial, thus connecting them together.

4. The needle is then taken to the other side and inserted from the superficial to the deep, forming another lock.

5. The loose ends are now tied together, forming a knot.

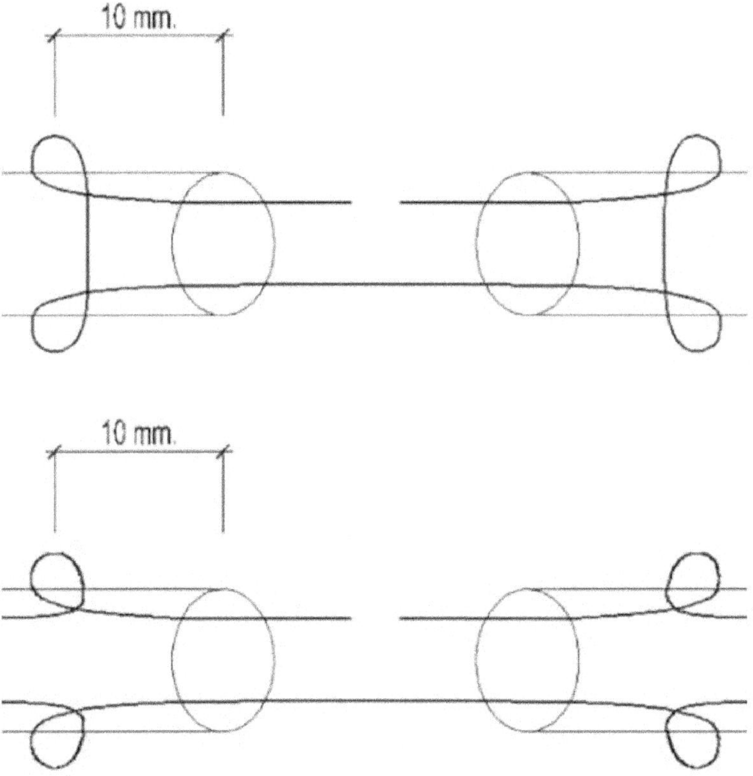

Cushing suture

This suture is primarily used to close the incisions in hollow organs such as the stomach, urinary bladder, and uterus. The suture penetrates the serosa, muscle layer, and submucosa (layer of connective tissue beneath the mucous membrane) without penetrating the organ lumen. This suture is an alternative to Lembert Suture.

Techniques involved include:

1. The needle is inserted perpendicular to and at a distance from the wound edge. It emerges from the deep to the superficial, a little further away from the apex of the wound.

2. It is then crossed over to the opposing wound edge and inserted at the same level. The needle takes a bite through the dermis and emerges a little further on the same side at the apex of the wound edge.

3. A knot is tied gently across the apex of the wound edge with the suturing material on either side of the wound edge. The short end is then cut off.

4. The needle is reloaded and oriented parallel to the incision line. On one side of the wound edge, the needle takes a bite through the dermis and emerges a little further away on the same side.

5. It's then crossed over to the contralateral side and inserted. The needle takes a bite through the dermis and emerges a little further away on the same contralateral side.

6. It's then taken back to the other side, inserted, and emerged a little further from the suture on the same side. It's then crossed again to the contralateral side.

7. This process continues through the entire wound length with the alternating needle sides.

8. At the end of the wound length, a reef knot is gently tied.

At the end of this process, it's observed that the wound edge is inverted and the knots buried.

The Running Pleated Suture

This technique is usually used when there's excess tissue created by the flap advancement. It's used to correct an imbalance in tissue length on two sides of a wound. This technique is designed to take advantage of forming multiple small pleats in the tissue that may be referred to as tiny Burrow's triangle all along the wound length leading to a shorter scar.

Techniques:

1. The needle is inserted at 90^0 to the epidermis of the wound edge, a little above the apex. It emerges on

the contralateral side of the wound edge on the same level as the initial insertion.

2. A knot is tied gently with the suturing material to avoid over constricting the wound edge. The short end is cut off.

3. The needle is then reloaded and taken to the wound length edge a little farther away from the suture knot.

4. A deep bite is taken at a distance farther away from the suture with the knot.

5. It is then rotated through the dermis and exits on the shorter wound edge at a point close to the suture knot.

6. The needle is crossed again over to the longer wound edge and inserted farther from the prior suture. A deep bite is taken through the dermis and rotated to the shorter wound edge, where it emerges close to the prior suture.

7. This process continues through the entire wound length, and a knot is gently tied with the loose ends of the suture material.

Frost Suture

It's a well-known surgical procedure for providing upward tension on the lower lid to prevent postoperative ectropion (turning outward of the lower eyelid). It's useful when there's a concern for postoperative edema. It's not to be used to correct ectropion that occurred during the operation.

Techniques:

1. After completion of closure, the needle is inserted through the tarsus or below it.

2. The needle takes a 3 mm bite and emerges at the conjunctival layer.

3. The needle is then reloaded and passed through the epidermis above the medial eyebrow keeping the lower lid in its anatomical position.

4. The suture material is then tied off gently to avoid over constricting the epidermis. The suture serves as a sling to suspend it and prevent eversion.

5. Adhesives strips can be used alternatively for positioning above the medial eyebrow.

Note: Suture placement in the medial lower eyelid must be done only by thorough familiarity to prevent damage.

The Bolster Suture

This is a niche procedure used for securing bolsters in place over the surgical site. Various bolsters secure skin grafts in place to enhance graft survivability.

Techniques:

1. The graft is secured in place. The needle is inserted at the 3 o'clock position perpendicular to the epidermis, tangential to the graft, 5 mm lateral to the graft edge.

2. The needle is rotated through the dermis, and the needle tip emerges at about 2-3 mm from the point of entry.

3. The free end of the suture may be held with a hemostat.

4. The suture is then similarly inserted at the 12 o'clock and 6 o'clock positions, respectively, with steps (1) and (2) repeated in each case.

5. The needle is passed around the suture material between the 9 o'clock and 12 o'clock positions.

6. Nonadherent dressing and gauze are cut to size and passed through the approximately 5 o'clock position placing them over the top of the graft in the desired position.

7. The ends of the suture material may be tightened by pulling up the ends toward the 3 and 9 o'clock positions.

8. A knot is then tied gently over the bolster.

CONCLUSION

A surgical suture, as you have learned, is a medical device used to hold body tissues together after an injury or during surgery. It is applied by using a needle attached to a thread. Several different sizes, shapes, and thread materials have been developed over its millennia of history. Dentists, surgeons, physicians, podiatrists, eye doctors, nurses, clinical pharmacists, and veterinarians, among other trained medical personnel, typically engage in suturing. Surgical knots are used in this process, and sutures generally can be classified into; Absorbable, Non-absorbable, Monofilament, Multifilament, and Barb Suture types. They are also differentiated in terms of size, material, usage, and coatings.

Understanding that the difference between you and the next great surgeon might just be anxiety and lack of practice is a step to becoming great at suturing.

Suturing might look hard but is easy, especially when you master the methods of this book.

Before You Suture

As a surgeon, there are certain words you should keep in mind while suturing;

Type of wound- Determine the type of wound to ascertain whether it can be sutured or not. Laceration, Abrasion, Punctures, and Avulsion.

Knots- Have a clear picture of the different types of knots available, including their techniques. Square knots, Surgeon's knot, Granny knots, Slip knots, Miller's knots, Aberdeen knot, Half-blood knot, Forwarder knot, Delimar knot, and Constrictor knot.

Aseptic techniques- Avoids breakdown of wounds. A surgeon must practice asepsis at all times. Use of antiseptics, hand washing techniques, carrying out major suturing in sterile fields, gowning, and donning of gloves.

Armamentarium- Get familiar with all instruments needed for suturing. Types of needles, needle holders, tissue forceps, artery forceps, scissors, dissecting forceps, etc.

Suture techniques- There are diverse suturing techniques needed to master the arts. The basic ones namely; Simple Interrupted Suture, Simple Running Suture, Vertical Mattress Suture, Horizontal Mattress Suture, Figure-of-8 Suture, Interrupted Cruciate Suture/Cruciate Mattress Suture, and the advanced ones, which are Hybrid Suture, Dermal/ Subcuticular Sutures, Purse-String Suture, Winch Suture, Cross Suture, Lembert Suture, Lattice Suture, Combined Vertical Mattress, Dermal Suture, Kessler's Locking Loop, Cushing suture, The Running Pleated Suture, Frost Suture, and The Bolster Suture.

APPENDIX:
Answers To Quick Exercises

Quick Exercise 1

1. B
2. A
3. Flexibility, Rigidity, Sharpness, Slimness.
4. End, Body, and Tip.
5. Straight Needle, Curved Needle, Half-Curved Needle.
6. A

Quick Exercise 2

1. A
2. A
3. A
4. Mayo scissors, Metzenbaum scissors, Iris scissors.

Quick Exercise 3

1. D
2. D
3. A
4. A
5. A
6. D

Quick Exercise 4

1. A
2. A.
3. A
4. A
5. C
6. Loop security, Knot security.
7. Square knot, Surgeon's knot, Granny knot, Slip knot, Miller's knot, Aberdeen knot, Half-blood knot, Forwarder knot, Delimar knot, Constrictor knot.

Quick Exercise 5

1. Treatment of underlying condition, Switch in medications, Avoidance of stimulants, Anti-seizure medications, Relaxation and Meditation, and Physical therapy.

2. A

3. A

4. B

5. A

6. Anxiety, Essential Tremor, Caffeine, Huntington's disease, Vitamin deficiency.

REFERENCES

Antony P., Tyle M.M., Mark D.W. and JR Soc. Med. (2011). History of suture journal of the royal society of medicine.

Carissa S., R.N. and Kristen C. (2021) Aseptic technique journal of medical line.

F.D Giddings. (2018). Surgical knots and suturing techniques. (5th ed.). Publisher: Giddings Studio Publishing. In

General Medical Disposable. Simple interrupted suture. https://gmdgroup.com.tr/en/simple-interrupted-suture/

Jayesh B.S., J.A., and Cerlif C. (2011). The history of wound care: Journal of the American College of certified wound specialists; 3(3): 65-66.

Micheal M. and Joseph A.M. (2021). Wound healing and repair.

M. Moastenbjork MD. And S. Meloni M.D. (2019). Suture like a surgeon: A doctor's guide to surgical knots and suturing techniques used in the departments of surgery,

emergency medicine, and family medicine. (1st ed.).
Publisher: Medical Creations. OSCE guide

Colin Brewster and Lain Anderson. (2021, January 8).
Simple interrupted suture: OSCE guide. Geekymedics.
https://geekymedics.com/simple-interrupted-suture-
osce-guide/

Sheen J.R. and Garla V. (2012). Fracture healing overview.
Method Mol Biol; 1130: 13-31.

Wayne W. LaMorte, M.D., Ph.D., M.P.H. Simple
interrupted stitch: Simple interrupted suture. B.U.
School of Medicine Surgery.
https://www.bumc.bu.edu/surgery/training/technical-
training/simple-interrupted-stitch/